I review over 100 books annually. This one is excellent! It captures the essence of being responsible with your own recovery. As a national TV host, I am bombarded with health books to review and comment on. I'd place this excellent book in the top 3 percent of every one I've ever reviewed. No better physician to report on true healing than one who has suffered from a life-threatening disease and not only lived but thrived after learning the truth and fixing himself. I highly recommend that you not only read this book, but, more importantly, heed this book.

—DOUG. A. KAUFMANN, HOST OF THE TELEVISION SHOW, *KNOW THE CAUSE*

If all American doctors practiced medicine like Dr. Becker then America would be a much healthier country and hospitals would be safer places to be. This book provides a compass to steer patients in the direction of lifetime health and toward the reversal of many chronic diseases.

—PATRICK QUILLIN, PH.D., R.D., C.N.S., DIRECTOR OF NUTRITION AT CANCER TREATMENT CENTERS OF AMERICA AND AUTHOR OF *BEATING CANCER WITH NUTRITION* AND FOURTEEN OTHER HEALTH BOOKS

As a practicing general surgeon, I found Dr. Becker's *Foundations for Healing* to be a clear, concise, yet thorough guide to superior nutrition. I plan to incorporate the information in my practice as well as in my own life. It seems that this important subject is too often presented only in the mass media. I recommend this publication as creditable food for thought and for life both in general and in specific.

—HOYT E. ALLEN, M.D., F.A.C.S.

Insightful and inspiring advice from a physician, using common sense to interpret scientific data for obtaining and retaining one's health.

—LEON WOLF, M.D. CLINICAL GASTROENTEROLOGIST

FOUNDATIONS *for* HEALING

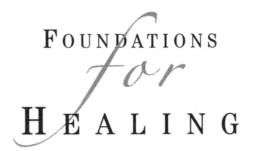

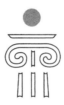

FOUNDATIONS *for* HEALING

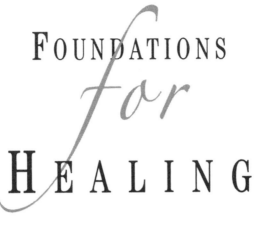

Holistic Plans for Your Return to

Health and Vitality

RICHARD L. BECKER, D.O.

BRIO PRINT

First Printing 2002
Second Printing 2003
Third Printing 2004
Fourth Printing 2005
Fifth Printing 2005
Sixth Printing 2006
Second Edition, First Printing 2006
Second Edition, Second Printing 2009

ISBN ISBN 0-9724656-0-X
LCCN 2002094479

BIO INNOVATIONS
P.O. Box 2485, Rockwall, Texas 75087
888.442.5150
www.bioinnovations.net

To Cindy, Tara, and Tana

who gave me a reason

to get well

CONTENTS
FOUNDATIONS FOR HEALING

1

Do not refer to this book for answers to medical questions or for the diagnosis of a medical condition—please see your doctor. Anyone with a health problem should discuss possible treatment with a qualified health care professional. The dosages listed in this book are meant to be a general guideline. Effective dosages vary from one person to another; discuss yours with a health care professional before implementing any recommended treatment.

ACKNOWLEDGMENTS

I want to thank my wife, Cindy, for her loyal support. She has been a loving wife and my partner in all things for twenty-three years. She has tolerated my shortcomings and given me the confidence to reach for the highest goals.

My daughters, Tara and Tana, have been a constant source of youthful enthusiasm. In addition they have given me the opportunity to think beyond my needs to those of others—and this is where true happiness lies.

Frank Jordan has been a mentor, friend, and confidant to whom I am indebted far beyond words.

I chose to emulate many of the doctors involved in my training, and I want to thank them here for their willingness to teach.

I would like to make a special acknowledgment to Doug Kaufmann, who helped me think on a grand scale and opened my eyes to a new way of helping people. Not only did Doug help nurse me to wellness, he allowed me to share my story with thousands.

To Dr. Victor Horadam, this special message: your kind manner and expertise in the field of oncology saved my life. Thank you! And to Tony Arterburn: when the times were tough, you were there for me every step of the way.

PART I

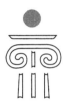

1

THE FOUNDATION

Declining health can sometimes leave us and our loved ones feeling overwhelmed. The amount of scientific knowledge today is staggering. You may be asking, "Who do I trust? Where do I start?" My life experience has taught me we must start with hope. Hope is as fundamental a human need as air and water. Do we not need confidence and trust? Do we not need the expectation that there is a way to make things better? Hope not only promises,

THE HUMAN SPIRIT NEEDS HOPE TO SURVIVE, BUT FALSE HOPE IS THE SHARPEST TOOL OF THE CHARLATAN.

it assures a better day is ahead. No matter what the condition, for the cure to succeed, hope must be present.

To hope, add the essential nutritional elements required for healing and sustaining life. The human species has nutritional needs that are undeniable and irrefutable. Just as hope provides a foundation for our emotional journey to wellness, our diet and nutritional supplements provide a foundation for our physical healing. When these elements are in place, the medicinal and surgical tools of our modern age can truly create miracles. I hope to offer you a sensible foundation for healing, unencumbered by statistics and scientific language. Pursuit of this knowledge and the application of it for the betterment of my fellow man has been one of my life's great joys.

A few years ago I traveled to a distant city to attend a medical conference seeking to advance my knowledge in the healing arts. I was excited when I learned that an expert in the field of preventive medicine was to lecture on advances in her field. This is truly a rare topic in a profession focused on disease and medical or surgical interventions. The entire hour was dedicated to immunizations, their indications, and potential side effects. No mention was made of the role that nutrition plays in preventing and treating disease, nor was anything mentioned of the benefits that every nutrition-minded person has come to know. The fundamental concepts embraced by the world of natural healing: diet, exercise, spiritual fulfillment, nutritional supplementation—all these were totally ignored by this world authority on preventive medicine.

I knew from that day forth that we cannot expect the established medical community to change the way we prevent and treat disease. Only the people of this nation have that ability, since throughout the history of our great nation all change for the better has come from them. When people demand it, doctors, the pharmaceutical industry, and others in the medical community will offer health care options that address the prevention, causes, and cures of disease.

Of the ten leading causes of death in the United States, eight can be combated by an intelligent program of healthy living. In our country, the treatment of disease has become a major challenge. The cost of medication has skyrocketed. The American people, who already pay more for health care than the people of any other country, have come to expect space-age medical marvels. Is more of the same the answer?

This book has been written as a guide that will serve as a foundation for healing. I hope to show how the most common conditions likely to arise in the realm of family medicine can be treated by natural methods. Patterns will emerge that will help correct a multitude of ailments—a regimen of prevention that can become part of your daily life. We all face the same diseases, but given a choice, why should we wait to contract them?

However, you may rest assured that in addition to helping you avoid unnecessary suffering on a day-to-day basis, should a time of crisis arise, a lifestyle of prevention will have provided you with a body that has been well-tuned to face and tolerate your medical and surgical options.

Though you may certainly use this book to look up a treatment for a specific problem, should you look a little further, you will notice that holistic treatments of common afflictions are similar. Despite similarities of treatment, however, holistic healing is not as simple as it might appear to the casual observer. If you look deeper, the patterns that will emerge in holistic healing will lead you to its fundamental truths.

In September 1997, I was diagnosed with Hodgkin's lymphoma. For the next three years, my family and I endured what thousands of cancer patients had before us. We were forced to put our lives in the hands of strangers, hoping they would make every effort to apply ALL their knowledge to my healing. I was amazed at how much of the cancer treatment was left to us. The treatment of the whole person was ours to implement.

From this crisis came healing and growth as a husband, a father, and as a doctor. I now know that the treatment of cancer and all disease involves much more than drugs, radiation, and surgery. The complete holistic treatment of disease includes all that God and nature provide.

I am now a member of a special club of cancer survivors. No amount of money or privilege will help one to gain entry. That can come only through prayer, faith, the grace of God, and daily efforts in all the aspects of healing. My first responsibility as a member in good standing is to help the next new member achieve what God and family have helped me to achieve—a second chance at life. I can truly say that cancer was one of the best things to happen to me. It has given me deep insight into the true nature of human suffering and shown me how to apply healing measures to those in need. In addition, it has given me the courage to stand up for what is right and what needs to be changed in American medicine today.

We all know there are fundamental truths in life, and that some are hard lessons to learn. Maturation takes time. The school of hard knocks will teach us some lessons. Careful observation of our peers will teach others. This process does not stop at twenty-one years of age or even at sixty-five.

It is a fundamental truth that doctors do not heal people. People heal themselves. A doctor, at best, may help you create an environment where healing may occur. It is a wise doctor who recognizes this truth and addresses the holistic nutritional needs of his or her patient. In addition, it is a wise patient who will accept his or her holistic nutritional needs and address them with each meal. Malnourished patients will not respond to the medical marvels of our age and will be forced to battle disease and aging with the most primitive methods.

To implement the measures outlined in this book will require courage. Courage is an attribute of character that often manifests itself as resolve and confidence. Courage is the foundation for change and a vital component of any plan for betterment.

It is also my purpose to devise a way of living based on the remarkably effective holistic measures used to treat common diseases. Preventive treatments can be incorporated in lifestyle practices, along with a manageable list of vitamins, minerals, essential fatty acids, proteins, and nutritional supplements. Why wait for a cure when the probability of one decreases with age, and when all conditions have a point of no return to vital health? It is the deeper purpose of this book to propose a lifestyle of holistic health and have you embrace its practices as fundamental truths.

THE COST OF TUITION IS HIGH, ESPECIALLY IF YOU DON'T GO TO SCHOOL.

Above all I hope you will embrace the truth that knowledge cures suffering. The statement found in Proverbs 11:9—"Through knowledge shall the just be delivered"—is as true today as it was thousands of years ago. Health and vitality will not come to you. You must seek them out.

2

THE PHILOSOPHY OF AMERICAN MEDICINE

In America most people do not think about their doctors' methods or philosophy. They simply think it is all about science and that whatever science proves, doctors will utilize.

Honestly, most doctors don't think about these things either. But we need to. Our patients' health and vitality—and our own—depend on knowledge and understanding.

A THEORY IS SOMETHING YOU BELIEVE IN WITH ALL YOUR MIND, BODY, AND SOUL; UNTIL YOU FIND SOMETHING BETTER TO BELIEVE IN.

The American system of medicine is historically based on a system of treatment called allopathy. Allopathy is defined by

Websters as "The system of therapeutics in which diseases are treated by producing a condition incompatible with or antagonistic to the condition to be cured or alleviated." Dorland's medical dictionary defines allopathy another way by stating, "Treat the symptom with an antidote." For example an antidote used over 100 years ago for snakebite was called Bibron's Antidote. It contained iodine, mercury, and bromine, all of which can be toxic when taken at high doses. Other antidotes included lithium carbonate to treat gout and lead to treat gonorrhea. Many of these early allopathic antidotes were poisonous and in some cases worse than the disease being treated.

Thank goodness, the antidotes of today are well-tolerated. Or are they? Let's say you have asthma and are taking steroids via an inhaler to calm your wheezing and labored breathing. The steroid compromises your immunity, so you contract a cold that develops into pneumonia. The pneumonia requires antibiotic treatment, which, in turn, gives you diarrhea and altered intestinal flora. The altered intestinal environment affects how you process and absorb the B vitamins in your food. A lower level of B vitamins in your bloodstream slows healing and causes an imbalance in the airway's smooth muscle metabolism, thereby causing more wheezing and necessitating another puff from the steroid inhaler. Unfortunately, we could create a scenario for each of the ten top-selling drugs in America just like the asthma scenario. Have we really advanced as much as we think?

I will be the first to admit that many of our antidote treatments of today are very effective for a variety of disorders. Also, I am not telling you to stop your medications. You must know, for the allopathic system to work, certain conditions must be present. First and foremost, this system assumes you are basically healthy. All you need is a little jump-start and off you will go, feeling great. Second, it assumes you are well-nourished.

Let me give you another example of how inadequate the allopathic system can be when the vital conditions of nourishment and basic health are not met. Let us say you are truly a healthy person who is bitten by a snake. You are also very lucky since you have been bitten by the snake in the hospital parking lot. You then walk into the emergency room to receive the antivenin and rest in a hospital bed for a day or two. Then doing well, you go home singing the praises of modern medicine. This is antidote treatment at its best!

Now let's suppose you are bitten by a snake while out in the desert. You have not had a proper meal in thirty days. You are sixty miles from the nearest hospital, and all you have for transportation is a slow-moving mule. Three days later you arrive at the emergency room. Your arm is swollen three times its normal size. You are delirious and close to death. You are malnourished, dehydrated, and have no reserves from which to fight. The antivenin will do you little good at this stage. The damage is done. You may lose your arm and maybe your life.

Now let's think about the antidotes for hypertension, cancer, infection, obesity, depression, and osteoporosis. Is the cancer patient fundamentally healthy? Are any of the people with these conditions healthy? They are basically and fundamentally sick. Is the antidote going to work? Too often it will not. Are you beginning to see the shortcomings of medications and the allopathic methods of care?

A MALNOURISHED PATIENT IS INCAPABLE OF RESPONDING FULLY TO MODERN MEDICAL AND SURGICAL PRACTICES.

What shall we do? Invent and take more and more medications at an ever-increasing cost? Frequently, such medications do not address the underlying cause of disease. Better medications are part of the answer, but to maximize health and provide cost-effective care in our country, we must become knowledgeable in the art and science of being healthy. You can leave the disease and its antidotes to the physicians. Learn from the lifestyles of the healthy. Eat every meal with your health in mind. Exercise regularly. Make a choice to be happy. Attain spiritual peace. Know your vitamins and supplements, and take them both as a cure and as prevention. Become familiar with the alternative health practitioners and know their long, productive history. Understand that the failures of modern medicine are our own in that we too often do not give the doctor a basically healthy patient to treat so that antidotes or corrective surgery may do their work.

3

BE YOUR OWN DOCTOR OF WELLNESS

Is it possible to integrate the best aspects of all the medical disciplines? Are we able to complement our current health care system with contributions from varied systems throughout the world? Yes, we can—in fact, it is imperative we do. To achieve this end, each person must become his or her own doctor of wellness. We all must learn the habits and patterns of the healthy and long-lived.

A PATIENT INVOLVED IN THE DECISION-MAKING PROCESS IS A PATIENT ONE STEP AWAY FROM WELLNESS.

In our computer age, knowledge is available to all who seek it out. The American system is but one method of healing. We must integrate healing knowledge from the entire scientific world. For this integration to work, it must have as its foundation a patient who is an active participant in his healing. He must also be knowledgeable in the practices and habits of the healthy.

The integration of alternative medicine into the American system is a daunting task. Still, many of the varied disciplines of science now contribute to the bank of knowledge used to treat and cure disease. The emphasis on prevention is imperative since, as the true causes of suffering are established, it has become increasingly clear that true cures for many diseases are in the distant future. Some time-honored natural remedies are being proven effective by modern scientific means, while ineffective ones are being discarded.

The financial impact on American medicine is undeniable, as big money interests drive the development of pharmaceutical agents and the education of American doctors. The influence of profit in health care, although capitalistic and American, slants our treatment regimens to the crisis and symptom alleviation mode by means of patentable drugs, which in many cases do little to correct the true reason for failing health.

Health insurance companies and government intervene in your health care decisions, taking the power away from you and your doctor, and setting standards of care that may not be in your best interest. The confidential conversations between doctor and patient are now being overheard by many sets of ears. Many wish to influence the decisions concerning your health without taking the ultimate responsibility for their failure.

Varying philosophies of treatment are as plentiful as carnies at a circus. Homeopaths, osteopaths, chiropractors, allopaths, naturopaths, to name a few, can be found in every city. Which works best? Whom can I trust? Everyone seems to profit from his or her point of view. When I really need help what do I do?

Have you ever heard the expression, "You can't be your own doctor"? Well, I am here to say that you must be your own doctor. Obviously, you can't remove your own appendix, but you can become more involved with your health care by understanding how to practice effective prevention in your daily life.

I had set out to write a short chapter on the integration of modern scientific medicine with traditional herbal and holistic nutritional healing. After much thought and introspection, I concluded that there is only one truth, one way to be healthy and to treat those who are sick. That is the ultimate discipline of science that includes the best of medication, surgery, vitamins, and herbal treatments, while also including homeopathy, osteopathy, physical medicine, acupuncture, and all the varied disciplines of allopathic medicine. Each facet is a part of the whole, which constitutes a complete method of healing. No one approach has an exclusive claim to the truth. The complete healer of the future will be well-versed in all.

At this point, you may be asking, "How can I possibly learn all there is to know about treating disease?" The answer is you can't. Even so, though there are a million ways to be sick, there are only a handful of ways to attain good health. The principles are the same for any race, culture, or ethnic background. The responsibility is yours to know what *healthy* is. The responsibility for diagnosing and treating your disease is your doctor's.

> THERE IS A DOCTOR OF WELL-NESS IN EACH AND EVERY ONE OF US. TALK TO HIM DAILY.

I firmly believe that if everyone spent just one hour a week in the study of healthy living, two hours a week exercising, and included a basic program of vitamin supplementation in their daily routine, the impact on alleviating human suffering would be tremendous.

The greatest challenge I have faced as a physician has been to implement a permanent change in the diet and lifestyle practices of my patients. When this is achieved, the results are impressive. I will now challenge my readers to study the preventive methods for healthy living, for this is truly the best cure of all.

4

THE BEGINNING TO THE END

For good health, fundamental requirements must be met. Though basic and applicable to all, these requirements are often overlooked resulting in our demise. Fresh clean air, abundant water, complete nutrition along with fulfillment of our psychosocial needs must all be accomplished if healing or the maintenance of vital health is to be expected.

Medical science has known for some time humans require specific nutrients or vitamins in their diets. In recent years it has been discovered during times of stress, illness or as a result of ageing the bodies level of certain metabolites, normally made by our body, drop to suboptimal levels resulting in the need to ingest these metabolites in our diet. These elements are called conditionally essential nutrients.

Modern science has also discovered the human body contains a wide variety of microbial life forms on our skin, our mouths and in our intestinal tracts that play vital roles in promoting health. These bacteria and the conditionally essential nutrients, in a normal, healthy setting are self sustaining; perpetuated by healthy dietary and lifestyle practices. (See Chapter 8 for discussions on the conditionally essential nutrients and probiotics.)

However when disease strikes or as aging takes its inevitable toll supplementing the conditionally essential nutrients and ingesting the microbial life forms that reside in and on our bodies become fundamental requirements for good health and healing. This is why the holistic physician believes the metabolic process of life begins and ends in the intestinal tract. The thirty feet of tubing (the intestines) is a complex structure responsible for extracting nutrient energy, vitamins, and minerals, along with the excretion of waste and toxins. The intestinal tract also plays a major role in our immune system as seventy percent of the immune system resides in the intestinal tract. An enormous diversity of potential immune-activating components, including pathogenic organisms must be screened, identified, and processed on a daily basis.

The upper intestinal tract is acidic and resistant to microbial growth; however, further down the intestinal tract, microorganisms are encountered in abundance. In the final three to four feet of intestines, the colon microbes, including bacteria, fungi, yeast, protozoa, and amoeba become the major constituents of stool, comprising half the stool weight.

A healthy intestinal tract, with a proper balance of microbes, is fundamental to good health. Without this delicate balance, health is always compromised. Any viable health-restoring plan must include measures to correct any intestinal dysbiosis (intestinal microbe deficiency or imbalance). This is where you must start your plan to better health.

In 1908, the Russian scientist, Elie Metchnikoff, wrote, "Ingested lactobacilli can displace toxin-producing bacteria, promoting health and prolonged life."[1] Metchnikoff won a Nobel Prize for these bold words. Today, Metchnikoff's legacy lives on in Russia and the worldwide scientific community. Much of our current research on the importance of healthy intestinal flora and the diseases an imbalance may cause has been done in Russia and other European countries. However in recent years American medical scientists have taken notice and they are also now contributing to this growing bank of knowledge. The following excerpts from various scientists' findings show this.

A. V. Valyshev showed that intestinal dysbiosis (altered intestinal flora) can cause inactivation of human leukocyte interferon, anti-lysozyme, and anti-complementary activity in apparently healthy and sick individuals, thus compromising the immune system and the ability to heal.[2,3,4] E. M. Gorskaia demonstrated that intestinal dysbiosis can cause an inhibition of the white blood cells called macrophages. The administration of probiotics (normal intestinal bacteria supplement) can reverse this suppression.[5] S. K. Kanareykina showed that ulcerative colitis patients (inflamed colon) had abnormal growth of proteus bacteria (intestinal dysbiosis), which causes inhibition of nutrient absorption in the small intestines, even though this area of the intestinal tract was not inflamed.[6] E. A. Lykova found that children with a variety of intestinal conditions, including allergies and infections, also had intestinal dysbiosis, resulting in an increase of bacterial endotoxins in their blood streams. This caused a significantly lowered level of intestinal antibody, Ig A, thus compromising their overall immunity. The researcher found the problem was correctable with the administration of probiotics.[7] Lykova also found that when children with intestinal dysbiosis contracted rotavirus, the most common cause of infant diarrhea, their illness lasted longer.[8] The Grabrichevesky Research Institute of Epidemiology showed that patients suffering from a variety of intestinal infections recovered faster if they took appropriate probiotics.[9] Z. E. Lineva showed that tuberculosis patients, receiving long-term antibiotics, developed intestinal dysbiosis with significant alteration of intestinal flora, which became worse the longer the duration of antibiotic therapy.[10] A. T. Akhmedov showed that children with lactose intolerance (inability to digest milk sugar) developed profound intestinal dysbiosis resulting in illnesses beyond that expected from just the inability to digest milk.[11]

In Czechoslovakia, the researcher, J. Kocian, found patients with dyspepsia (indigestion) from radiation therapy, poor digestion, or antibiotic therapy responded favorably to the administration of probiotics, significantly shortening the time of recovery.[12]

Researchers in the United Kingdom showed that elderly patients have a significant alteration of their intestinal tract microbes. The researchers suggested that correction of this imbalance could improve the health of senior citizens.[13]

In Bulgaria, a study found that chronically constipated patients showed a significant propensity to develop intestinal dysbiosis.[14] The same conclusion was met in an Italian study of children with chronic constipation.[15]

In a study reported in 1986, twelve patients with food sensitivities and intestinal dysbiosis attained significant reduction of food reactions when their dysbiosis was corrected with probiotics.[16]

A German study revealed that of 314 patients sick from a variety of illnesses, 55 percent showed upper intestinal dysbiosis. If patients suffered from a pancreatic disease, 64 percent showed upper intestinal dysbiosis.[17]

A study conducted at the Tripler Army Medical Center found a correlation with intestinal dysbiosis and chronic venous insufficiency.[18]

In a review on attention deficit/hyperactivity disorder in *Alternative Medicine Review*, the authors concluded that nutritional treatment of attention deficit/hyperactivity disorder, including the correction of intestinal dysbiosis, favorably improved treatment outcome.[19]

Studies also show that live-culture yogurt with Lactobacillus acidophilus is more effective in preventing recurrent candida vaginitis than pasteurized yogurt.[20]

It seems everyone is now concerned about their LDL-cholesterol levels. Recent research shows probiotic therapy is even capable of significantly lowering LDL-cholesterol levels.[21]

The British Medical Journal reports children who were given a probiotic nasal spray are less likely to develop recurrent otitis media (ear infections) after an initial course of antibiotics.[22]

The American Journal of Clinical Nutrition reports women who eat foods containing probiotics like yogurt at least three times a week were 80 percent less likely to develop urinary tract infections than women who consumed probiotics less than once per week.[23]

A recent unpublished study conducted by the Mitsubishi International Food Ingredients in North America finds seniors over 65 who supplemented probiotics and took an influenza vaccine showed lower rates of influenza, higher influenza antibody titers, required fewer antibiotics and displayed an improved immune response compared to seniors who just took an influenza vaccine.

While research was being conducted for the first edition of this book the National Institutes of Health Medical Library (www.pubmed.gov) contain approximately seventy research articles relating to intestinal dysbiosis and probiotic therapies, today the number of articles far exceeds three-thousand. There is no other area of medicine that holds greater promise for those in failing health.

The above list is a short representation of the research conducted since Elie Metchnikoff's original work in 1908. A full review convinces the diligent student of the profound effect an altered intestinal microbe balance can have on health and the critical importance of correcting the imbalance in those who are sick from seemingly unrelated illnesses.

What is needed for those who are sick is a complete plan to correct the imbalance of intestinal dysbiosis. Is taking just a probiotic enough to attain optimal health? My experience has taught me that a probiotic alone is not enough to create a lasting health benefit. One must also include a diet that restores this delicate, health-promoting intestinal microbial balance, a diet that provides maximum nutrition and health restoring elements, essentially a diet that heals.

5

THE BIBLICAL DIRECTIVE,
A STARTING POINT
FOR GOOD HEALTH

To each life comes times of suffering, despair and soul searching. If health challenges complicate these troubling times we often feel confused and powerless; unable to understand what is wrong or what changes should be made so our mind, body and spirit may return to wholeness. If you face these challenges, as a physician I recommend you embrace the basic and fundamental dietary and lifestyle practices discussed in this book. As a patient who has battled cancer, I recommend if you are facing troubling times, return to your spiritual roots and embrace them once again. Just as when Malachi wrote of the coming of the prophet Elijah during a time when Elijah would...

*"...restore the hearts of fathers to their children,
and the hearts of the children to their fathers..."*

Malachi 4:6

so should we return to our spiritual roots during our quest for better health.

The Bible is a most impressive book; containing wisdom, knowledge and history. It not only offers advice for spiritual enlightenment but it also provides guidelines for dietary and lifestyle practices that will help restore your health and vitality. The Bible, as a historical document, can help you understand our ancestral way of life. The way of life that helped the human race succeed and flourish. Understanding our historical ways is of utmost importance as modern times have presented us with a wide variety of lifestyle and dietary options –many of which are a detriment to our health and well being. Modern scientific investigation has validated the wisdom of the Biblical Directive for a long and healthy life making the Biblical Directive a starting point for your healing. The holistic physician proclaims the mind, body and spirit must be in unity for vital health. For you to succeed in your quest for better health, you too must acknowledge and embrace this fundamental need for unity.

The first Biblical reference to diet is found early in the Book of Genesis thus underscoring diet's vital role in our health.

> *"And God said, See, I have given you every herb that yields seed which is on the face of all the earth, and every tree whose fruit yields seed; to you it shall be for food."*
>
> Genesis 1:29

The Hebrew word for herb is eseb –a word with many definitions including green, grass, tender shoot or herb. By understanding the Hebrew definition of eseb it becomes clear that nature provides us with a wide variety of plant based foods to not only sustain us but to assure good health well into our senior years. If interpreted in a broad sense this powerful verse identifies three basic vegetarian sources of nourishment for mankind –herbs, fruits and vegetables. Perhaps the most precious pearl gained from this verse is the implication that we should include a variety of fruits and vegetables in our daily diet. Far too often we eat the same fruits and vegetables day after day. Dietary variation assures complete nutrition.

Water flows throughout the Bible as it is mentioned over 700 times. It is perhaps, the substance most commonly used to portray a spiritual meaning. In the Bible water metaphorically represents physical birth, the gift of life, the word of God and

God's ability to purify, spiritual fulfillment, everlasting life and even a source of eternal grace and salvation. The first reference to water is found in the book of Genesis.

"Then God said, "Let the waters teem with swarms of living creatures, and let birds fly above the earth in the open expanses of the heavens."

Genesis 1:20

This verse underscores the vital importance of water in our health: Water is the source of life and must it be consumed in abundance or disease and death will follow.

The Olive tree and its fruit is a Biblical and universal symbol of peace and rebirth and its oil was used for food and spiritual anointing. This special tree lives longer than any other tree creating a symbolic figure for a source of everlasting life and renewal. When Noah wanted to see if the waters of the great flood had abated he sent out a dove.

"And the dove came to him toward evening; and behold, in her beak was a freshly picked olive leaf. So Noah knew that the water was abated from the earth."

Genesis 8:11

The ancients relied upon the olive tree, its fruit, oil and its leaf. Bread was made with olive oil. Herbs and medicinal tinctures were formulated with olive oil. The fruit could be salted and preserved for a future meal and the leaf was used as a medicine. It is hard to imagine the lives of the Children of Israel with out the olive tree. Modern scientific investigation validates the ancient's reliance on this special gift of nature. The Mediterranean Diet, touted as cardiovascular health promoting, relies heavily on this special plant.

Among the plant based foods wheat holds a position of dependability and sustenance in the Bible. It was considered a staple in Biblical times as it is today. Psalm 147:12-14 and Joel 2:23-24 proclaims a bountiful wheat harvest is a blessing from God to His people. The New Testament, in John 12:24, uses wheat as a symbol for the death and resurrection of Christ. Christ's last meal contained bread made from wheat. Barley is also held in high Biblical esteem. Mentioned almost 40 times, barley metaphorically represents a prophet or the one who comes first to announce the Messiah. Barley is also often used to portray a new beginning –a fresh start. However today's food products that contain wheat and grain are often altered beyond recognition. The refinement of grains, a common food preparation practice in the modern world has significantly compromised grains' nutritional value. If you include grains in your diet make them whole grains, just as they were consumed in Bible times. Scientific investigation has validated the practice of eating whole grains as healthy food beyond any doubt.

Perhaps the food that held the highest level of symbolic importance was the grape and its juice as it was frequently consumed during times of celebration and religious ceremony. Hundreds of passages portray the grape as a symbol of fruitfulness and the New Testament uses grape juice or wine as the symbol of Christ's blood. The ancients maintained vineyards for hundreds of years passing them down generation to generation and many of them are still producing a harvest today. The very fact a grapevine can produce fruit for such extended times implies one of the grapes most remarkable health benefits –longevity. When you eat a handful of grapes your body is benefiting from the powerful antioxidant, resveratrol. It is found in grape skins and numerous studies have shown that this amazing substance may prolong life while helping to prevent cancer. The ancients did not have the benefit of modern scientific investigation yet they knew what was good for them!

The authors of the Bible chose the fig tree and its fruit, a delectable nutrient packed super food, to portray the overall health and well-being of the Children of Israel along with peace, rest and strength.

"And Judah and Israel dwelt safely, every man under his vine and under his fig tree."

1 Kings 4:25

"Do not be afraid, ye beasts of the field: for the pastures of the wilderness do spring, for the tree beareth her fruit, the fig tree and the vine do yield their strength."

Joel 2:22

In Matthew 24:32-33 when Christ was asked about signs of His second coming He states, "Now learn the parable from the fig tree: when its branch has already become tender, and puts forth its leaves, you know that summer is near; even so you too, when you see all these things, recognize that He is near, right at the door." We can be assured, only a plant that bears a fruit of the highest value would be used to portray such important events and sentiments. Today the fig is most often consumed as a sugared cookie –a far cry from its historical use and elevated role.

The pomegranate, a fruit most of us have never eaten, is given a unique distinction in the Bible as being closely linked to the House of God –not once but twice. When God was giving Moses directions for the tailoring of the garments to be worn by the priests He stated,

"And you shall make on its hem pomegranates of blue and purple and scarlet material, all around on its hem, and bells of gold between them all around: a golden bell and a pomegranate, a golden bell and a pomegranate, all around on the hem of the robe."

Exodus 28:33-34

Hiram, skilled in bronze work and one of the builders of the Temple of Solomon used pomegranate figures to adorn the capitols atop the bronze pillars used to support the Temple roof.

"So he made the pillars and two rows around on the one network to cover the capitals which were on the top of the pomegranates...and the pomegranates numbered two hundred in row around both capitals."

1 Kings 7:18-20

What we now know about the health providing benefits of pomegranate does nothing to diminish its historical status. Pomegranate is an excellent source of antioxidants, fiber, vitamin C and it plays a critical role in maintaining prostate health in men. It is unfortunate the pomegranate is the least consumed fruit in North America.

The lentil, perhaps the most nutritious legume and an excellent source of protein, was a prevalent, highly prized food in ancient times. Esau was willing to sell his birthright for some bread and lentil stew.* King David and the Children of Israel were willing to defend their lentil fields with their lives.

> *"...And the Philistines were gathered into a troop, where there was a plot of ground full of lentils, and the people fled from the Philistines. But he (David) took his stand in the midst of the plot, defended it and struck the Philistines; and the Lord brought about a great victory."*
>
> 2 Samuel 23:11-12

Lentils, when combined with wheat provide complete protein, capable of sustaining even an army. It is no wonder David made his stand there in his prized lentil field.

The Bible goes on to name several more foods; almonds, spelt, milk and honey to name the most commonly mentioned. Since the almond tree is the first tree to bloom in the Holy Land, it is seen as a sign of new hope and rebirth. Almonds are an excellent source of protein, vitamins, minerals and omega-3 fatty acids. Spelt is a hardy grain, resistant to disease and infestation. It has a

*Genesis 25:34

rich nutty flavor and is a good source of B vitamins. Milk and honey are held as reward for a job well done or a source of rejuvenation after a long journey.

> *"So I have come down to deliver them from the power of the Egyptians, and to bring them up from that land to a good and spacious land to a land flowing with milk and honey..."*
>
> Exodus 3:8

This attitude toward honey —one of reward is an attitude we should adapt. We should not make sweets a part of our daily diet. Yet from time to time the "sweet tooth" strikes and we are compelled to have a treat. When this happens make your treat honey. Even small amounts will satisfy a sweet craving; a feature unfound in the sugar and corn syrup based treats that are so common today.

The Bible also clearly defines the animal based foods the Children of Israel should eat. These foods are labeled as "clean" meats. Moses and Aaron were given these specific instructions:

> *"Speak to the sons of Israel, saying these are the creatures which you may eat from all the animals that are on the earth. Whatever divides a hoof,*

thus making split hoofs, and chews the cud, among
the animals, that you may eat."

Exodus 11:2-3

Animals having these characteristics –chews their cud
(ruminants) and a split hoof, include: sheep or mutton, cattle,
goat, deer, elk, antelope and buffalo or bison. We now know
these animals carry few parasites and the meats of these
animals are resistant to spoilage. Also the fat of these animals
contains lower levels of saturated and trans-fats than pork and
other forms of "unclean" meats.

The dietary guidelines for fowl are also clear. Exodus
11:13-19 provides a list of birds that should never be
eaten; they include birds that are either carnivores,
flightless or scavengers. These types of animals harbor
huge numbers of putrefying bacteria and are prone to
parasite infestation.

Perhaps the Old Testament guidelines for the consumption of
fish are the most insightful of all.

"These you may eat, whatever is in the water: all that
have fins and scales, those in the water, in the seas or
in the river, you may eat."

Leviticus 11:9

Fish with fins and scales have the highest content of the health providing and cardiovascular disease preventing omega-3 fatty acids of any fish or sea food, plus their protein and vitamin content is unparalleled.

The Bible provides guidelines for use of substances that may inebriate us –advice that has been too often ignored in times of old and in the modern world.

> *"So then do not be foolish, but understand what the will of the Lord is. And do not get drunk with wine for that is dissipation, but be filled with the Spirit."*
>
> Ephesians 5:17-18

The Old Testament even provides dietary guidelines for times of extreme conditions such as may occur during wilderness survival, war, famine or prolonged migration.

> *"Yet these you may eat among all the winged insects which walk on all fours: those which have above their feet jointed legs with which to jump on the earth. These of them you may eat: the locust... the devastating locust... the cricket... and the grasshopper... But all other winged insects which are four footed are detestable to you."*
>
> Leviticus 11:2-23

Let us hope we never have a need to eat these insects but if conditions are severe and survival is in question, the Bible has told us which insects we may eat and not become sick from the meal.

Ponder now for a moment the important roles these Biblical foods fulfill –both spiritual and physical. Would the authors of the Bible choose to fulfill these roles with substandard unhealthy foods?

HAPPINESS IS BEST PURSUED BY ALWAYS
CHOOSING TO DO THE RIGHT THING.

6

THE HEALING DIET

For thousands of years, humans have sought to better themselves by fasting. When Moses was called to lead his people out of Egypt, he went to the desert and fasted. Clarity of mind and purity of body was essential for the job at hand. All the world's great religions have a history of fasting to improve both mind and body.

Modern science has explained in part the benefits and risks of such endeavors. We know that when the body is deprived of food its chemistry changes. After the blood's sugar or glucose has been depleted from the liver and muscles, the body begins to burn fat stores for energy. The transition from glucose metabolism to fat metabolism can be

THE MORE THINGS CHANGE, THE MORE THEY STAY THE SAME.

difficult to endure. The body's system does everything in its power to compel us to eat. Hunger, weakness, fatigue, and irritability drive us to find another meal. If the meal is delayed, and we must call upon our adipose tissues (fat) for energy, remarkable changes inevitably occur. The appetite diminishes, energy abounds, and mental clarity is returned. By the very existence of the fat-burning metabolism, nature has provided the means to find another meal. If we must hunt and gather for our next repast, this newfound sense of purpose created by burning fat is clearly to our advantage. Our entire system is placed on red alert. Senses are activated. Wound-healing is accelerated. Immunity is heightened.

Science tells us that if we continue to fast, with no caloric or nutrient intake whatsoever, our metabolic rate will begin to slow. We must conserve our energy resources to survive. The essential protein needed for daily production of blood, immunoglobulins, and enzymes is taken from our muscle and organ stores. The water-soluble vitamins are depleted within a week, and our system becomes critically depressed. This taxing condition creates adrenaline and stress hormones that suppress our immunity. Death is inevitable if starvation continues beyond forty days. Clearly, complete and prolonged deprivation of nutrients is no way to heal.

Science has also taught us how to harness and perpetuate the initial phase of fasting, during which time the appetite is numbed, energy is increased, healing and immunity are accelerated, and there is heightened mental clarity. All these benefits can be sustained by depriving our systems of just the sugars, starches, grains—carbohydrates—while continuing to ingest protein, low-starch vegetables, low-sugar fruits and berries, and fats and oils, along with the essential vitamins and minerals.

Before you conclude this as a new fad diet that will go away, consider this. Harry Truman once said, "The only thing new is the history you don't know." The history of disease is a part of the academic curriculum of all doctors. The history of nutrition is not. Serious students of the human condition must seek this knowledge on their own.

Through the ages, humans have had no means of preserving food past the season of harvest. Not until comparatively recent times have salting of meats, storage and refinement of grains, and the canning of fruits and vegetables been available for use. When the grain was harvested in the fall, it was consumed quickly before it could spoil. The autumn harvest's high-starch meal added pounds of energy reserves, increasing the likelihood of surviving a hard winter.

Those of you who grew up or live on a farm have witnessed this phenomenon time and time again. You have observed farm livestock gain weight on grain and silage to prepare them for winter's challenges. Humans also show this propensity to gain weight when fed a high-starch diet. Our primitive ancestors had no means to preserve, store, or grow sufficient grain to last an entire year. Nor could they include sweet fruits and berries in their everyday diets, for these would spoil if not eaten immediately. But modern man has solved this dilemma by increasing grain yield through hybridization and modern farming techniques, along with the preservation of grain by refinement and preservatives. Now, modern man can eat a high-starch diet for as long as he wishes. He can consume fruits and vegetables out of season by means of canning, freezing, and rapid transportation from distant growing fields. Today's consumer can eat from around the world without traveling farther than the local grocery.

Although this recent historical development has its advantages and conveniences, it is inconsistent with the habits and practices of food consumption that brought the human race to its present state. It is still common practice to eat only "in season" in most of the world today. This "in season" food consumption practice is consistent with our historical diet and allows cycles of partial fasting that are of great benefit to our health. One need not be deprived of high-starch meals for months at a time to benefit. A weekly cycle of food variation will suffice for the healthy. More prolonged starch- and sugar-avoidance cycles are required for those with chronic illness. Their cycles should more closely resemble those of our natural dietary history.

The typical American diet today, featuring fast and prepackaged foods retains little of our ancestral dietary roots. Today's teenagers and young adults have been raised on sugared cereals, pizza and hamburgers, while water has been replaced by a super-sized soft drink. Far too many mature and senior adults have also succumb to the convenience of America's new-found dietary practices, a practice that must be corrected if a return to vital health is expected.

There is nothing more frustrating for patient or doctor than to be told by a panel of experts that "there is nothing to cure this condition." I, like many, have refused to accept this dismal prognosis. It is our duty to continue our efforts even if it seems futile, just as Job continued though he had lost all. By understanding and combining the dietary practices of our ancestors with the scientific knowledge of our brilliant researchers, and with the dedicated caring of our medical professionals, hope has been restored for many of the desperately ill. People are winning the battle with cancer on a daily basis. Systemic lupus erythematosus, rheumatoid arthritis, depression, heart disease, and many other pathological conditions have miraculously gone into remission when this diet is used as a foundation for healing. Know that it can happen. Believe that healing is within your grasp. Make a change in your life for healing today. Know that the longest journey to vital health begins with your decision to make your daily dietary lifestyle a part of your healing.

There are several important points that you should consider prior to initiating the HEALING DIET. The successful patient consistently adheres to the following rules:

Rx _____

POINTERS FOR SUCCESS

1. Eat a wide variety of allowed foods. Avoid a limited diet.

2. Eat at least two servings of allowed fruits and berries daily.

3. Drink one-half ounce (1/2 oz) of chlorine-free, filtered tap or bottled water per pound of body weight daily.

4. Do not be afraid to eat meat but choose lean organic meats whenever possible. They will not raise your cholesterol while on this diet. The fat will be burned for energy; however, it is wise to limit red meat fat by cutting away any excess and/or choosing lean cuts.

5. Emphasize fish and eggs, as they are high-quality foods. Do not drain the oil off tuna as this oil has tremendous healing properties, even if it is an added vegetable oil.

6. Eat mixed raw nuts and seeds, both as a snack and as part of a meal.

7. If you have an initial "healing crisis," eat allowed fruits, berries, nuts, and seeds, along with a large glass of water and you will feel better soon. (See Chapter 7—THE HEALING CRISIS.)

8. Eat large garden fresh salads, featuring a diversity of greens, with a variety of colored vegetables and copious amounts of olive, walnut, hazelnut and flaxseed oils.

9. Breakfast "is served" within one-half hour of rising in the morning. If you do not care for traditional breakfast foods, you are not required to eat them.

Eat any of the foods allowed, but never skip this meal. Breakfast is critical to your healing and maintaining your ideal weight.

10. Eat at least three meals and one snack daily.

11. If you have gained weight during your decline in health, continue the HEALING DIET until near your ideal weight. The pace of weight loss should be slow, generally no more than two to three pounds per month overall. Fast weight loss is stressful and is rarely permanent. The first month of the diet will result in a five- to fifteen-pound loss for men and a three- to ten-pound loss for women. This initial rapid weight loss should not be expected to continue.

12. If you have gained weight a low-sugar meal replacement product may be used to replace 1 or 2 meals or as a snack daily. (See Chapter 23—OBESITY.)

13. If you have not gained weight during your illness, maintain your weight with meat, poultry, fish, eggs, nuts, seeds, and oils.

14. Continue the HEALING DIET until you attain a pattern of vitality. This means you feel well on a daily basis. It is normal to become fatigued after a

week of work or activities. However, a day or two of rest should restore your good health. It is also normal to become tired when you catch a cold or flu. A few days of rest should restore you. If a cold or flu puts you to bed for two weeks, your health has not been restored. You should continue the HEALING DIET until daily vitality is restored.

15. Once you have attained a consistent sense of well-being, advance to the TRANSITIONAL DIET by gradually introducing TRANSITIONAL DIET foods into your dietary routine. If this change of diet makes you feel unwell return to the HEALING DIET. If you are tolerant of the gradual introduction of new foods, make the transition complete and start following the TRANSITIONAL DIET. Pay close attention to your body's reaction to newly re-introduced foods as food allergies and sensitivities may be playing a major role in your declining health.

16. While on the TRANSITIONAL DIET, you may combine any legume (bean) with a whole grain for a complete protein source, as many people tire of meat.

17. Once your vitality has been maintained on the TRANSITIONAL DIET, you may progress to the DIET FOR THE REST OF YOUR LIFE.

18. The entire process, from starting the HEALING DIET to starting the DIET FOR THE REST OF YOUR LIFE, may take up to three years. Many patients feel apprehensive when they are told the length of time required to attain wellness, fearing that their success with the program will be threatened if they can never eat many of the foods they love for such a long time. One of the most remarkable results of this dietary plan is the consistent change people make in what they consider good food. Eventually, refined and sugared foods will not appeal to you! And if you do eat poor quality foods in the future, your body will tell you immediately that you have made a mistake.

Richard L. Becker, .D.O.

THE HEALING DIET

MEATS – All meats are allowed, including beef, pork and ham (limit intake), veal, lamb, mutton, liver, goat, buffalo, and venison. Processed, salted, cured meats and pork are allowed but should be limited, including sausage, bologna, bacon, salami, jerky, frankfurters, and hot dogs.

POULTRY – All poultry is allowed, including chicken, turkey, pheasant, quail, dove, goose, guinea hen, pea fowl, prairie chicken, Cornish hen, and duck.

FISH – All fish are allowed, including salmon, cod, halibut, tuna, sea trout, fresh water trout, sole, sardine, haddock, herring, orange roughy, red snapper, mackerel, king fish, sea bass, freshwater bass, swordfish, mahi mahi, scrod, shark, catfish, pike, crappie, perch, bluegill, bream, and flounder.

ORGANIC FOODS ARE THE MOST NUTRITIOUS FOODS. EAT THEM WHENEVER POSSIBLE.

CRUSTACEANS – All crustaceans are allowed; however, they should be limited to one serving per week, including lobster, prawns (shrimp), crab, and crayfish.

MOLLUSKS – All mollusks are allowed; however, they should be limited to one serving per week, including clams, oysters, scallops, escargot, squid (calamari), and mussels.

EGGS – All types of eggs are allowed, including chicken, turkey, duck, and goose.

DAIRY – Only the following dairy products are allowed: 100% pure butter, 100% pure cream, sour cream, cream cheese, cow and goat milk yogurt (plain, without pre-added fruit or sugar), cottage cheese, and buttermilk. No "light" or fat-reduced dairy products allowed.

OILS – Include any of the following oils as a food or supplement: flaxseed, hemp, fish, olive, borage, primrose, lecithin, safflower, soybean, sunflower, grape seed (excellent for frying and cooking), walnut, hazelnut, black currant, pumpkin seed, sesame seed, canola, and perilla.

VEGETABLES – All low-starch vegetables are allowed, including the following:

asparagus, broccoli, Brussels sprouts, carrots, cauliflower, celery, chicory, cucumbers, dulse, eggplant, endive, kelp, nori, kombu, and all types of seaweed, mushrooms, okra, onions, leeks, parsley, peppers, radishes, sprouts, tomatoes, watercress, olives, cabbage (all types, including sauerkraut, red, green, kale, and Chinese),

greens (all types, including beet, chard, mustard, kale, dandelion, spinach, and turnip),

lettuce (all types, including butterhead, bibb, Boston, celtuce, iceberg, lamb's, matchless, oakleaf, prize head, salad bowl, red leaf, chicory, arugula, and romaine),

squash (all types, including acorn, alligator, banana, boston marrow, buttercup, butternut, caserta, cocozelle, Connecticut field, cushaw, delicious, golden nugget, hubbard, mammoth, mirliton, pumpkin, Quaker pie, Queensland, straightneck, table queen, turban Virginian, whitebush scallop, and zucchini).

FRUITS – Only fresh or fresh frozen tart fruits and berries are allowed, including the following: lemons, limes, grapefruit, Granny Smith apples, avocados, blueberries, raspberries, hackberries, huckleberries, cranberries, blackberries, strawberries, boysenberries, pomegranates and kiwi fruit.

NUTS AND SEEDS – All fresh raw nuts and seeds or butters derived from nuts and seeds are allowed, including the following: almonds, pecans, walnuts, Brazil nuts, cashews, hazel nuts, pignolia nuts, sunflower seeds, pumpkin seeds, and squash seeds.

WATER – Consume 1/2 oz per pound of body weight of filtered or bottled water daily.

BEVERAGES – Coffee in moderation is allowed. You may use 100 percent cream in your coffee. Tea is preferred—black, white, or green. Carbonated mineral water, unflavored, and unsweetened is also allowed.

SWEETENERS – Stevia is allowed.

SPICES – All spices are allowed.

VINEGAR – Use only unpasteurized apple cider vinegar as a supplement or as a salad dressing.

JUICE – Juice from any fruits or vegetables listed including carrots.

FOODS NOT ALLOWED ON THE HEALING DIET

SUGARS – All sweet substances, refined or otherwise, are prohibited, including sucrose (white table sugar), corn syrup, maple syrup, honey, molasses, maltose, dextrin, mannitol, fructose, or any sweet substance, no matter the source.

GRAINS – All grains whole or refined are prohibited, including wheat, bulgur, barley, oat, rye, rice, pasta, corn, quinoa, buckwheat, corn chips, potato chips, cereals of any type—whole grain or refined, breads of any type, and tortillas of any type.

VEGETABLES – Those with arthritis and autoimmune diseases should avoid the nightshade group of vegetables, including tomatoes, potatoes, eggplant, and peppers.

LEGUMES – All legumes are prohibited, including beans – black, pinto, kidney, and red – black-eyed peas, English peas, soybeans, green beans, lentils, chick peas, split peas, garbanzo beans, and peanuts.

STARCHY TUBERS – Potatoes, yams, sweet potatoes, turnip root, and beets.

DAIRY PRODUCTS – All dairy products except those listed in allowed foods are prohibited, including milk, skim milk, half-and-half, cheese of any type, and goat's milk.

FATS, OILS, AND ADDITIVES – Lard, margarine, hydrogenated fats and oils, aspartame, MSG, and food colorings.

CARBONATED BEVERAGES – All carbonated beverages except unflavored, unsweetened mineral water are prohibited, including sugared and artificially sweetened soda.

PICKLES AND VINEGAR SALAD DRESSINGS

ALL ALCOHOLIC BEVERAGES

THE TRANSITIONAL DIET

Add to the HEALING DIET the following foods:

GRAINS –All grains are allowed in the whole grain form such as oats and oatmeal (long cooking variety), wild rice, brown rice, rice milk, wheat germ, whole grain wheat flour tortillas, quinoa, millet, amaranth, buckwheat, whole grain breads, and cereals without added sweeteners, such as bulgur breakfast cereal and granola.

VEGETABLES – Add the low starch nightshade group of vegetables as tolerated, including tomatoes, eggplant, and peppers.

DAIRY – Organic cheeses from cows or goat milk as tolerated.

FRUITS – All fruits are allowed with continued emphasis on the tart fruits and berries with gradual introduction of the sweeter fruits, including oranges, tangerines, figs, plums, cherries, apples, peaches, grapes, and pears.

LEGUMES – All legumes and beans are allowed, including lentils, peas, black-eyed peas, pinto beans, black beans, soy products, soymilk, soy cheese, and peanuts.

Continue to avoid corn, sweet substances, refined white flour breads, pastas, potatoes, yams, and white rice while on the TRANSITIONAL DIET.

THE DIET FOR THE REST OF YOUR LIFE
Add to the TRANSITIONAL DIET the following foods:

SUGARS AND SWEETENERS – Honey, molasses, pure maple syrup, rice syrup, and brown sugar in moderation as tolerated.

FRUITS – All fruits previously listed are allowed with the addition of papaya, pineapple, mango, and melons. The HEALING DIET fruits may be eaten all year. The sweet fruits and melons may be eaten frequently during their season of harvest; when out of season, they should be eaten only occasionally.

VEGETABLES – All vegetables are allowed. Include daily consumption of raw vegetables. Beets, yams, and sweet potatoes may be added in moderation as tolerated. White potatoes should be eaten infrequently.

GRAINS – All grains are allowed in the whole grain form, including whole grain pastas, vegetable derived pastas, and whole grain breads. However, do not eat grains every day.

DAIRY – Reduced fat organic milk is allowed if tolerant of milk.

FOODS TO AVOID FOR THE
REST OF YOUR LIFE

Any prepackaged, highly processed foods should be avoided, including sugared or artificially sweetened soft drinks, potato and corn chips, sugared cereals, cookies, candies, cakes, and pastries. Refined grain foods such as pasta, white rice, and white bread should be avoided. Avoid corn syrup, white sugar (sucrose), maltose, dextrin, mannitol, fructose, aspartame, and MSG in your daily diet.

Continue to avoid cow's milk, if intolerant, and nonorganic cheeses.

Continue to avoid corn in your daily diet.

Continue to limit the intake of processed, cured, and salted meats, including bologna, bacon, sausage, salami, jerky, hot dogs, and frankfurters.

After completing the dietary progressions, you will have learned much about food and its effect on your health. Exclude any food that compromises your health from the DIET FOR THE REST OF YOUR LIFE. For example, if tomatoes and peppers aggravate your arthritis, do not include them in your diet.

You may have occasional treats, such as pasta dishes and desserts, but they can never become a daily part of your diet. This will be of less concern than you may think, for your tastes will change.

As you re-introduce foods into your diet pay close attention to your body's reaction to these foods as food allergies and sensitivities may be playing a major role in your declining health.

7

THE HEALING CRISIS

If you come down with the flu, your body tells you to rest. If you are dehydrated and need fluid, you become thirsty for a drink of water. If you have been working hard and then become weak, your body tells you food is needed. At the end of a long workweek, your body tells you to take the weekend off for rest. It is intuitive to listen and to do all these things. Over time we learn that the price of ignoring our body's signals is high. If we continue to ignore the warning, the price of recovery is higher than if we had responded promptly.

SOMETIMES IT MAY GET WORSE BEFORE IT CAN GET BETTER.

When health declines gradually, our body's messages may be misinterpreted and an improper, unhelpful response may follow. I want you to be aware of an unusual syndrome of failing health called Pica syndrome. Pica describes an abnormal craving for and eating of foods or substances not normally part of our diet, such as dirt, clay, chalk, starch, or ice—when the patient is profoundly iron-deficient. These substances actually bind iron in the intestines, preventing its absorption and making the iron deficiency worse. This unfortunate person's internal messages have become unreliable, driving him or her to destructive measures in the futile attempt to correct a nutritional deficiency. No medication will stop this behavior. Only iron will correct the problem.

Consider the patient with fibromyalgia and chronic fatigue. This person has utter exhaustion as a constant companion. Her entire body aches, her mind is depressed, and her sleep is fretful, never improving her complaints. She props herself up with frequent caffeinated drinks, sweet snacks, muscle relaxants, and pain pills. She may also take a sleeping pill in hopes that her sleep will be more rewarding. Eventually, depression sets in and antidepressants follow. Her weight slowly increases from her lack of exercise and poor dietary habits. Do you see the pattern of false body messages? Is this person really any different from those with pica, those who eat dirt when anemic? If iron deficiency can cause such abnormal behaviors, can other nutrient and body system deficiencies perhaps cause similar syndromes? She may not be iron deficient, and she may not display the classic behaviors of pica, yet she certainly shows the tendency to engage in feeding and symptom-alleviating behaviors that will not cure the condition.

The allopathic doctor will ask about her symptoms and prescribe an antidote. The holistic physician will ask what happened in her life, perhaps many years ago, which changed her pattern of vitality. Did she require frequent or prolonged antibiotics for acne, or an ongoing sinus or bladder infection? Was she under prolonged stress, such as that which occurs in a stormy marriage? Did delivery of three babies in a four-year period deplete her body of vital nutrients?

These are questions that must be answered before a proper healing plan may be implemented. However, when the corrective plan is begun a strange and confusing phenomenon may occur—the HEALING CRISIS. The unfortunate patient begins to feel worse than ever! The fatigue is amplified, the joints scream in revolt, and the depression is overwhelming.

Have you ever gone to bed with the flu and had a terrible night? You soak the sheets with sweat and have disturbing dreams. Early in the morning the fever breaks and you awaken, feeling like a new person, free of the misery that sent you to bed in exhaustion. You have experienced a HEALING CRISIS. Your body has gone to war in an effort to thwart the disease agent.

Unfortunately, in chronic afflictions the healing crisis may last for several weeks. For the sufferer of such conditions, if by chance they may stumble upon an effective treatment for their condition and thereby initiate a HEALING CRISIS inadvertently, every fiber of their being tells them to stop what they are doing, even if it is the only thing that can bring about healing!

Let me explain this in another way. Imagine you are in a huge warehouse with twelve grand pianos all perfectly tuned. You strike middle C firmly on the center piano. As a result, every middle C piano wire in the warehouse will begin to vibrate. If, while C is sounding, you then strike C sharp, discord occurs; not only does it hurt your ears and sense of melody, the previously vibrating middle C strings and C sharp strings all abruptly stop. Health and disease states have vibration energy just as middle C and C sharp. When effective disease treatment is implemented, health discordance often occurs, inflicting initial suffering just like our example of musical discord.

Before you conclude this is just a new-wave, hocus-pocus, fast-talking scam, understand that the magnetic resonance imaging tests used today to visualize internal organs is based on this same concept. Normal tissues have a specific vibration of magnetic energy, and abnormal or diseased tissues have different energies. The computer scanners sense the difference, and the radiologist interprets the picture generated by the computer as a disease entity.

DESPITE THE RELENTLESS EFFORTS OF OUR LAWYERS, POLITICIANS, AND HEALTH INSURANCE EXECUTIVES, THOSE WHO HAVE CHOSEN TO CARE FOR THE NEEDS OF OTHERS ARE STILL DOING SO.

When healing begins to occur, it is frequently accompanied by a healing crisis. As you start the HEALING DIET, the most important part of your plan, be prepared for initial challenges. You may feel dizzy, weak, and/or in need of a sugar fix. Your joints may ache and a different type of depression from what you are accustomed to may temporarily overcome you. In general, a worsening of the symptoms you are trying to eliminate occurs. If the healing crisis strikes, eat some berries, a Granny Smith apple, a handful of nuts, drink a large glass of water, and take a rest. You will feel better in time. The feeling may return, but rest assured, it will pass.

8

NUTRITIONAL SUPPLEMENTS

Nutritional and agricultural experts report the nutrient quality of our foods has diminished due to modern farming techniques. This phenomenon requires us to supplement our diet with the essential vitamins and minerals for healing and the maintenance of vital health. During my years of clinical practice I have observed countless patients recover from

JUST BECAUSE IT IS NOT A PRESCRIPTION DOES NOT MEAN IT IS INEFFECTIVE.

baffling syndromes of failing health when they simply added a smart supplement plan to their healthy diet.

CONDITIONALLY ESSENTIAL NUTRIENTS

In recent years medical scientists have also discovered during times of stress, failing health or as a side effect of medication our bodies may be unable to make certain key metabolic compounds that are responsible for a variety of essential functions. For example during cancer therapy the livers' ability to produce Co enzyme Q10 may be compromised leading to decreased energy flow to the heart resulting in cardiomyopathy or even heart failure. The list of conditionally essential nutrients is quickly expanding as our understanding of this vital concept is becoming more complete. The conditionally essential nutrients such as Co enzyme Q10, L-carnitine, D-ribose, L-arginine, L-glutamine and lutein are important supplements to include when appropriate for your health recovery. Many of the supplements recommended in part II of this book are conditionally essential nutrients.

NATURAL ANTIBIOTICS

Throughout human history infectious disease has taken more lives and caused more human suffering than any other single cause and this simple fact remains true even today. The invention of antibiotics certainly has played a role in stemming this tide of suffering; however, antibiotic therapy comes with a long list of side effects including disturbance of the sensitive intestinal microflora.

Prior to the invention of probiotics, herbs and plant extracts were commonly used as antimicrobials. Their use today is still applicable as long term therapy while these natural agents have very few side effects and they do not disturb the flora of the intestinal tract. Oil of oregano, olive leaf extract, Pau d Arco, grapefruit seed extract among others have been studied and proven effective for the long term management of chronic infectious processes such as chronic yeast and candida infections. Most syndromes of failing health have at their root some form of infectious disease. Including these natural antibiotics in your treatment course may be of great benefit to your health.

PROBIOTICS—
Micro-Organisms that Promote Good Health

The discovery that bacteria and other microscopic life forms are capable of causing infectious disease has dramatically changed the way humans live. Herculean efforts and huge sums of money have subsequently been dedicated to public sanitation and scientific research on how to prevent and treat the diseases these microscopic agents are capable of causing. The typical household reflects microbial awareness with cleansing agents, antiseptics, antibiotics and a dramatic change in daily hygiene practices –changes aimed at destroying these virulent agents and preventing the diseases they may cause.

The discovery that germs cause disease has truly changed us. Although the breakthrough has lead to the ability to treat and prevent many diseases and overall better living conditions it has also lead to a presumption that all bacteria and microbes are bad. This erroneous conclusion has in turn lead to delays in our understanding of the role normal intestinal microbes' play in our health and their therapeutic benefit when ingested during times of illness or as a means of preventing disease.

Humans are born with a sterile, microbe free intestinal tract. The first health promoting microbes (probiotics), particularly Lactobacillus acidophilus, are introduced to the infant through contact with mother's breast and her milk. As raw foods are introduced the intestinal microbes begins to diversify; as a child's dietary diversity advances so does the diversity of the intestinal microbial ecosystem. Over time diet provides the child and subsequent adult with a continuous source of probiotic intestinal microbes. A diverse diet, complete with raw and fermented foods such as yogurt, has historically provided an ample source of these critical beneficial microbes. However with scientific advancement and the justified fear of germs it has created has come a significant change in the quantity and type of beneficial probiotic bacteria contained in our foods. Milk is pasteurized. Yogurt is pasteurized. Our foods contain preservatives and they are frequently irradiated, further destroying any remaining probiotic organisms. Vegetables are sterilized and canned. We are under constant stress and we travel to the four corners of the earth. Our water supply is chlorinated and we take antibiotic medications –all these things have a profound affect on the quantity and quality of our intestinal microbial residents.

These factors and more make it imperative we have an assured continuous source of these life-giving intestinal probiotics, in our daily diet and as a dietary supplement. If only these basic biological concepts could be understood and put into practice, many who are suffering an endless cycle of illness could be helped. The simple act of eating health food store quality yogurt, buttermilk, kefir, sour cream, raw fruits and vegetables along with taking a daily dose of a high potency probiotic supplement all are fundamental to good health. They remain one of the most powerful therapeutic tools for the treatment and prevention of disease available today.

Even a cursory review of the proven health promoting attributes of probiotics convinces the most ardent skeptic of their merit. During the course of writing the first edition of this book in the year 2001 the National Institutes of Health's Medical Library –PubMed, contained only about 70 scientific writings that discussed the varied role our intestinal microbes play or the health promoting benefits of taking probiotics.

Today the number of articles far exceeds three-thousand. Our knowledge in this critical area is growing by leaps and bounds. The table below lists some of the more common probiotic organisms and few of their proven health benefits. Take a moment to review the table; the knowledge gained will help you understand why eating foods that contain probiotic organisms and taking probiotics supplements are fundamental to good health. For up to date probiotic information visit the website www.pubmed.gov and search for the specific probiotic organisms. What you will learn may change your life!

LACTOBACILLUS ACIDOPHILUS

- Promotes effectiveness of blood stream white blood cells

- Increases circulating blood antibodies

- Binds to and lowers intestinal content of carcinogens

- Lowers the incidence of vaginal infections including those due to candida

- Makes an antibiotic like substance (lactocidin) that protects from and shortens the course of bacterial intestinal infections (food poisoning)

- Produces vitamin B 12

- Lowers LDL cholesterol

- Produces lactase thereby improving lactose intolerance

Bifidobacterium bifidum

- Promotes effectiveness of blood stream white blood cells
- Increases circulating blood antibodies
- Reduces the incidence and severity of infant diarrhea
- Enhances the assimilation of dietary minerals
- Lowers blood pressure
- Helps to regulate body weight and blood glucose
- Suppresses the growth of Helicobacter pylori, a cause of stomach ulcers

Lactobacillus helveticus

- Promotes mineral absorption and the formation of bone
- Promotes intestinal pH balance by producing lactic acid
- Reduces the incidence of kidney stones
- Inhibits the growth of fibrosarcoma and colon cancer
- Promotes muscle recovery after exercise
- Reduces blood pressure

Bifidobacterium longum

- Produces molecules that bind minerals turning them into anti-oxidants
- Reduces antibiotic associated diarrhea
- Lessens the production of fecal toxins
- Improves circulating antibody levels

ENTEROCOCCUS FAECIUM

- Reduces antibiotic associated diarrhea

- Lowers LDL cholesterol

- Protects from travelers diarrhea and intestinal viruses

- Improves absorption of B vitamins

LACTOBACILLUS PLANTARUM

- Makes an antibiotic like substance (bacteriocin) that protects from and shortens the course of bacterial intestinal infections (food poisoning)

- Reduces the occurrence of infections after intestinal surgery

- Synthesizes the amino acid L-lysine promoting immunity to herpes virus

- Produces nitric oxide thereby promoting immunity and circulation

- Reduces antibiotic associated diarrhea

- Creates nutrients used by intestinal cells

LACTOBACILLUS RHAMNOSUS

- Reduces symptoms of eczema

- Reduces symptoms of allergic rhinitis, asthma and food allergies

- Reduces the incidence of bladder and kidney infections

- Increases the phagocyte activity of macrophages (white blood cells)
- Suppresses inflammation

LACTOBACILLUS SALIVARIUS

- Freshens breath
- Deters tooth decay
- Increases circulating interferon
- Helps to prevent intestinal inflammation

THE ESSENTIAL FATTY ACIDS

The discovery of abandoned children who have been raised by dogs has revealed, if a child grows up in an environment devoid of human contact and communication, the child will not be able to develop normal cognitive and communication skills throughout life. This remains true even if they receive intensive therapy upon placement into an environment rich with human contact. The full impact of childhood neglect is just now becoming fully understood. Humans have long recognized we need nurturing during childhood to attain our fullest potential in adulthood. Just as we have psychological needs for growth and development, our bodies require certain key dietary elements in order to achieve our fullest physical potential and to promote healing and vital health.

The science of nutrition is a relatively new science. It was not until the early 1900's that scientists uniformly began to question what molecules in food are absolutely essential for life. It had been obvious to all that lack of food led to death. Early nutritional scientists also observed individuals who consumed enough calories yet they still became ill and perished if a change of diet was not implemented. From this humble beginning a huge bank of powerful knowledge has evolved. Today most of us are aware our diet must contain key elements or dire consequences are sure to follow. What remains to be acknowledged by the majority is that even though life can be sustained with a poor diet, overtime the substandard diet greatly accelerates aging and disease processes. It is a detriment to humanity that so many of us, doctor and patient alike, remain unaware of this potentially life saving acumen.

Over the last century much has been learned about nutrition. Perhaps the most powerful knowledge gleaned is the understanding of the role essential fatty acids (EFAs) play in our health. The essential fatty acids are food oils required in the diet. They can not be made from other dietary components and must be present in our foods. The essential fatty acids are alpha-linolenic acid, an omega-3 fatty acid and linoleic acid, an omega-6 fatty acid. The denotation omega-3 or 6 tells us where in the molecule a double bond between carbon atoms occurs. The EFAs are also called poly-unsaturated fats. There are several other dietary oils that have similar omega-3 or omega-6 configuration but differ in other respects that can be adequately substituted for the two original EFAs just as there are several forms of vitamins C, D and E. The chemistry of the EFAs is complicated but if you can just remember, we need a daily source of omega-3s and omega-6s in our diet and which foods and supplements contain them, you will hold powerful knowledge.

We now know the EFA omega-3s and omega-6s play a variety of critical roles in normal physiology and the prevention of disease. The EFAs provide the building blocks for strong cell walls. The EFAs are turned into molecules that promote healing after injury. They calm the ever present tendency toward inflammation, swelling, fever and pain. If an infectious agent invades us the EFAs help activate the immune system. They help regulate our hormonal system. They stabilize blood sugar. They increase energy, athletic performance and stamina while promoting muscle strength and deterring muscle breakdown. Our brain's chemical network also turns the EFAs into substances that create a mood of quiet, satisfied calm. They even influence our genetic code's ability to relay our blue-print of individual uniqueness along with the code for healing and wellness. The most impressive role of the EFAs is their ability to prevent the accumulation of arterial plaques thereby preventing cardiovascular disease –the leading cause of death in America.

There is another type of omega fatty acid. They are the omega-9 monounsaturated fatty acids. Although not an essential nutrient they do provide health benefits. The most common omega-9 fatty acid is oleic acid and its consumption has been shown to help prevent heart disease and diabetes. Omega-9 fatty acids are a common dietary component consumed by cultures that reside around the Mediterranean Sea.

The types of fats that are harmful when consumed in abundance are the trans fats and the saturated fats. These types of fats are unfortunately very tasty and they provide abundant calories. The trans and saturated fats feed physiologic enzyme processes that counter the health benefits of the omega-3s and omega-6s. They promote obesity, cardiovascular disease, arthritis and inflammation, premature aging and cancer.

A quick review of common foods and their varied fat content reveals to even the casual observer America consumes too much saturated and trans fats. This practice has lead to a major deleterious health effect. You will notice some foods are listed under multiple headings. This is because the foods contain a variety of fats and oils. Also the saturated and trans fat category contains some foods that are relatively healthy foods. These foods are best consumed in moderation and in their low or non-fat form.

In order to assure the essential fatty acid dietary requirements are fulfilled I recommend you frequently eat the foods listed that contain the omega-3s, 6s and 9s along with supplementing the omega-3, 6 and 9 nutrients so you are assured their daily requirements are met. Too achieve this goal I recommend you take fish oil or flaxseed oil with borage oil: 1-6 grams of each daily.

Foods Containing Omega-3 Essential Fatty Acids

Flaxseeds

Cold Water Ocean Fish
including: Salmon, Mackerel, Sardines, Anchovies, Tuna

Walnuts, Almonds, Brazil Nuts

Pumpkin Seeds, Sesame Seeds

Soy Beans

Wheat Germ

Dark Green Leafy Vegetables
including: Kale, Spinach, Mustard Greens,
and a variety of Dark Green Lettuces

Foods Containing Omega-6 Essential Fatty Acids

Flaxseeds, Grapeseeds, Borage Seeds,
Evening Primrose Seeds, Black Current Seeds

Pine Nuts, Pistachio Nuts, Walnuts, Almonds, Pecans

Sunflower Seeds

a variety of Meats, Poultry and Seafood

Foods Containing Omega-9 Non-Essential But Health Promoting Fatty Acids

Olives and their Oil, Sesame Oil

Avocados

Almonds, Pecans, Cashews, Peanuts, Hazelnuts, Macadamia Nuts

Foods Containing Large Amounts of Saturated (S) and/or Trans (T) Fats

Hydrogenated Vegetable Oils (T)
(common ingredient in prepackaged and fast foods),
Margarine (T), Shortening (T), Butter (S+T), Coconut Oil (S),
Cottonseed Oil (S), Palm Kernel Oil (S), Corn Oil (S),
Peanut Oil (S), Safflower Oil (S)

Cream and Cheeses (S+T)

Pork Fat and Lard (S+T)

Whole Milk (S+T)

Saturated and Trans Fats are present in a less damaging form in the
fat of all meats including beef, mutton, venison and poultry

VITAMINS AND ESSENTIAL MINERALS

The human body with its complicated workings is the pinnacle of creation. No man made machine can compare with the complexities contained within each and every one of us. Further it is a marvel that life is capable of sustaining itself and even correcting itself (healing) even when aberrations (disease) occur. And it all happens with no conscious effort... or so we assume.

Modern times have brought many conveniences and improvements resulting in a standard of living that has never been equaled. Here in America we produce so much food we are capable of feeding many of the world's less fortunate with our surplus. And since this battle to attain our high quality of life required many generations' hard work and sacrifice it is only natural to assume that the dietary and lifestyle practices we have retained would only be of the highest quality. But unfortunately this is not the case.

With affluence comes complacency and with the accumulation of abundant food, goods and assets, comes an inevitable devaluation of these item's true worth. Simply stated the dietary and lifestyle practices that have lead to the success of America are now being abandoned by those who are benefiting the most from the hard work of our forefathers. We must do everything in our power to retain the time tested, health promoting dietary and lifestyle practices of the past while incorporating quality-of-life advances into our daily lives. In short we must always be aware of the true value of the "dietary and lifestyle dollar".

One of the greatest concerns expressed by today's nutritional experts is the value, or the vitamin, mineral and overall nutritional worth of our foods, is eroding. It is not hard to imagine that America's favorite meal –a fast food hamburger, fries and a soda, has less nutritional value than a prime cut of lean beef, fresh vegetables, whole grain bread and a garden salad. It is also not hard to imagine that a plot of land that once produced forty bushels of wheat per acre but is now capable of producing over two hundred bushels per acre may now produce wheat that is not as nutritious as the lesser harvest. We are all aware of the economic and market driving forces that have placed the highest priority on food volume, appearance and taste over food's nutrient quality. And we have come to accept the abundant, tasty and cheap versions of food as a hallmark of progress and equivalent or superior to our traditional ways. But they are not. And their acceptance as nutritious has lead to the development of vitamin or mineral deficiencies in over fifty percent and obesity in over sixty percent of the American population.

If you are struggling with your health it is unwise to assume you are free of any vitamin, mineral, amino acid or essential fatty acid deficiency. The healing of the human body –with all its varied aspects accomplished without any apparent thought, is completely dependent on meeting these critical-nutrient-needs. The majority will be capable of meeting these needs by eating a diet rich in fresh organic foods and by supplementing high quality multiple vitamins, minerals, amino acids and essential fatty acids. Some will require the administration of vitamins by intravenous or intramuscular injections but they are the minority. I strongly recommend you include a multiple vitamin preparation in your plan of recovery and subsequent plan for prevention of disease. Do not assume your needs are being met.

Always take your vitamins and minerals with food and a large glass of water. If taken on an empty stomach with little fluid, nausea and indigestion are sure to follow. In their natural state, vitamins are found in foods complete with fiber and buffering agents. Taking them alone, on an empty stomach can be very irritating. If breakfast is typically a light meal, take your vitamins after supper but include them in your plan for they are fundamental to your recovery.

We all live in a fast paced world with schedules that require, from time to time, we take repast from modern food sources.

The practice of taking a daily multiple vitamin will help assure you are not among the Americans who are nutrient deficient —now the majority, while providing you with every nutrient needed for healing and vital health.

When you go to the health food store looking for a good supplement you may find row after row of vitamin- and supplement-filled shelves offering a thousand options. It is overwhelming; there are so many choices. Which brand is best? What is the correct dose? Do the health food store clerks really know what they are talking about? These are all valid questions. A little advice could make this all-important decision-making process a little more comfortable. Consider the following when making vitamin, mineral, and supplement purchases.

Rx _____

SUPPLEMENT GUIDELINES

1. If you have a laboratory or physician confirmed deficiency of any essential element, replace that element with a product that features only the deficient element as an active ingredient, along with a separate multiple vitamin. For example: if you are diagnosed with iron-deficient anemia, take a product with just

iron as its active ingredient to assure the requirement is met. Add to the iron product a multiple vitamin and mineral preparation for completeness and full absorption of the deficient element.

2. The Reference Daily Intakes (RDIs) established by the Food and Drug Administration refer to the minimum amount of nutrient to prevent vitamin deficiency states and are not enough to promote vital health.

3. Vitamins, minerals, amino acids, and essential fatty acids work in concert. Too much of one can be as dangerous as not enough.

4. Avoid combination products that feature multiple herbs. If you have a bad reaction, you will not know what you are reacting to. Also combination products that feature multiple herbs frequently underdose various certain ones, compromising their effectiveness. If you find a helpful combination of individual herbs, you can then combine these in one product at the proper dose. This is a particular problem in soy phytoestrogen products that contain multiple herbs. Keep this type of supplement as simple as possible.

5. Powder, capsule, gel-caps, and liquid supplements are generally better than hard-pressed pills. The pill forms do not dissolve and absorb as well as the others. They can also create highly irritating concentrations of vitamins as they dissolve in the intestinal tract. However, pills are the most convenient to take. If a liquid or powder form of a supplement tastes terrible to you and you are considering stopping it altogether, change to a capsule form and follow the instructions on the label to avoid side effects.

6. Unless otherwise instructed always take your vitamins, minerals, and supplements after a full meal and with a large glass of chlorine free water. Nature always provides fiber and other nutrients with vitamins and minerals. Taking these supplements on an empty stomach causes nausea and limits their effectiveness.

7. The very best multiple vitamin and mineral products feature chelated elements. This is achieved by combining the vitamin or mineral with an essential amino acid protein carrier or Krebs cycle molecule that buffers the essential nutrient and promotes slow, even absorption. The Krebs cycle is the normal physiologic process by which we chemically derive

energy from glucose. Aspartate, citrate, fumarate, malate, succinate, oxaloacetate, acetyl, and alpha-ketoglutarate are all components of the Krebs cycle and capable of safely attaching to essential nutrients and slowly releasing them for absorption in the intestinal tract.

8. Use only food source natural vitamins and minerals.

9. When choosing an herb or herb extract, look for products that contain standardized active components. This standardization reflects quality control.

10. Do not shop for supplements based solely on price. Ask the attendant his or her experience with the product. Find out if it sells well due to happy repeat customers.

11. Vitamins, minerals, supplements, and herbs should be treated with the same respect as medication. You can get too much of a good thing. A single plant may contain hundreds of different chemical compounds. Taking too many herbs or supplements can be as dangerous as taking too many medications. Do not use mega dosages without the supervision of a heath care professional.

12. Avoid supplements that are promoted through marketing techniques that do not disclose the exact content of the supplement. For example: some products are promoted on television as being effective for the relief of arthritis pain yet the ads do not reveal what the product contains. You must be fully aware of what you are paying for and ingesting at all times.

13. Develop a relationship with your health food store attendant. The knowledge and experience of such people can be very helpful.

14. Obtain a reference book such as the *Physicians' Desk Reference for Nutritional Supplements* to provide reliable information to help guide your supplement choices.

15. Inform your physician and pharmacist of all your supplements, even if they do not ask. In general, anything you can buy at a health food store is well tolerated and does not interact with medications; however, there are a few exceptions.

Richard L. Becker, .D.O.

9

POLYNESIAN NONI
MORINDA CITRIFOLIA

Throughout the ages, people have tried to better themselves by the use of herbs, tinctures, and natural remedies. Each successful culture has time-proven natural remedies that are relied upon for healing and the relief of suffering. One of the most powerful tools of natural healing is the wondrous tropical plant *Morinda citrifolia*. The Polynesians call this gift of nature Noni. The Noni plant grows in tropical regions around the world, and it thrives in volcanic soil near shore under the elevation of 1,300 feet.

EVERY SUCCESSFUL CULTURE HAS AT LEAST ONE NATURAL HEALING REMEDY THAT MAY CONTRIBUTE TO YOUR GOOD HEALTH.

There is a 2000-year recorded history of medicinal use, including all parts of the Noni tree, from roots to flower petals. But the most prized and powerful part of the plant is the juice of the fruit. The scientific community is currently studying this remarkable plant in an effort to fully explain what the ancient healers of Polynesia, the kahunas, have known for thousands of years: *Morinda citrifolia* has amazing healing abilities.

Dr. Annie Hirazumi of the Department of Pharmacology, John A. Burns School of Medicine, University of Hawaii, conducted an experiment to see if *Morinda citrifolia* has anticancer effects. A genetically induced, cancer-susceptible strain of mice was divided into two groups. The first group was injected with aggressive lung cancer cells and fed a normal diet. The second group was injected with lung cancer cells, as the first group; however, they were given Noni juice as a part of their diet. Among the first group of mice, all died of cancer with none surviving longer than twelve days. The Noni-fed mice all survived for at least twenty-four days, and nine of the twenty-two Noni-fed mice survived for fifty days or longer.[24]

In a study conducted by the Department of Pathology, University of Illinois College of Medicine, Rockford, researchers found that rats given cancer-causing agents were 30 to 90 percent less likely to show signs of cancer, depending on the organs examined and the sex of the rat, if given Noni juice before and after the cancer-causing agent.[25]

A team of Japanese researchers studied the extracts of over 500 plants, searching for anticancer phyto-chemicals (plant-origin chemicals). They determined Noni was the most effective anticancer plant of all the plants tested.[26]

A French group of researchers wanted to determine if *Morinda citrifolia* has analgesic properties (pain relief). They found Noni to be nontoxic and to "show a significant, dose-related, central analgesic activity in treated mice," with no evidence of dependency forming substances.[27]

A Clark Atlanta University research team showed a *Morinda citrifolia* extract inhibited the growth of the disease causing fungi Candida albicans and Aspergillus nidulans confirming Noni's role in controlling chronic yeast and fungal infections.[28]

A Coreana Skin Science Research Center of Korea study reveals *Morinda citrifolia* stimulates the productions of collagen and normal human fibroblast confirming Noni's role as a wound healing and skin beautifying agent.[29]

From an unexpected yet greatly appreciated letter to the editor of the European Journal of Gastroenterology & Hepatology, Dr.

Claude J. Jensen and fellow researchers report *Morinda citrifolia* helped protect laboratory animals from liver damage when they were exposed to known liver toxins such as carbon tetra-chloride. This information is good news as agents proven to protect the liver are sorely lacking. Our ever expanding list of liver transplant recipients attests to this fact.[30]

In a study conducted by Dr. Mian-Ying Wang, 85 percent of the people who took Noni juice for a total of thirty-three different conditions stated their condition was improved by the addition of Noni to their diet. Neil Solomon, M.D., Ph.D., surveyed over 15,000 Noni juice drinkers and found that 80 percent had both subjective and objective improvement of various health conditions.[31]

One must ask how could any one thing be so helpful for so many? It is almost too good to be true. The current scientific thinking is that Noni juice, with its special combination of natural components, helps to normalize cell function by its ability to improve DNA-directed protein and enzyme production and function. This goes to the very core of life itself, as we are the sum of tens of thousands of enzyme-controlled chemical reactions. Pain is relieved, mood is lightened, clarity of thought is improved, energy is restored, and the body's weight is normalized over time when Noni juice is added to a sensible wholesome diet.

Ralph M. Heinicke, Ph.D., has found Noni juice to be rich in the chemical and enzyme complex called bromelain. According to Dr. Heinicke's research and writings, two of the components of the bromelain complex are called xeronine and proxeronine. Xeronine is the component of the bromelain complex that helps to normalize DNA-directed protein production. However, xeronine is unstable and quickly degrades when the Noni fruit is processed into juice. Fortunately, according to Dr. Heinicke's theory, proxeronine is stable and is readily converted into xeronine in the intestine by another enzyme component of the bromelain complex called proxeroninase. Nature has provided a wonderful delivery mechanism for a remarkable healing substance, xeronine, which modern science has yet to replicate.[32]

Pineapple was at one time an excellent source of bromelain, but modern agricultural techniques have dramatically reduced the pineapple's bromelain and xeronine content. Noni juice has forty times more xeronine than pineapple, making it nature's most reliable source of this soothing substance. I believe there is more to Noni than just the bromelain complex. In fact, the newest research suggests Noni juice's polysaccharide component may play a vital role in improving health.[33]

Polysaccharides are complex chemical structures and are known to play a role in the immune system's communication network. They have been shown to safely and effectively activate and normalize immune function. Nature has given us an entire natural "medicine cabinet" in the small package of Noni juice, with over 170 plant chemical components creating a symphony of natural healing and with a 2000-year history of safe use.

Although the Noni plant is hardy and grows wild without cultivation, the delicate balance of special ingredients in the fruit juice is fragile. Noni juice does not withstand processing, reconstituting, and high temperatures needed for complete pasteurization used in various Noni products available today. To receive the maximum benefit from Noni juice, consume only fresh juice or potency-proven concentrate.

The taste of Noni juice is startling and repugnant, so many companies dilute their Noni juice products with sugar and sweet fruit juices. Avoid these products, as we ingest enough sugar without adding it to our supplements. I have talked to hundreds of fresh Noni juice drinkers, and most tell me that they adjusted to the taste of pure, fresh juice with time, and many admit they look forward to their Noni dose as they associate the benefits of this supplement with its potent taste.

You may add some grape juice, as you choose, to help you grow accustomed to the taste.

I urge you to include the juice of pure, fresh *Morinda citrifolia* in your plan for better health. Start with just one ounce of Noni juice a day on an empty stomach, followed by a full glass of water. If your condition has not improved after two weeks, increase the amount to two ounces daily. The vast majority of Noni juice drinkers will see a benefit to their health with one to three ounces daily and within sixty days. There is no upper limit in dose, and large quantities such as a quart a day have been used for the treatment of cancer, as a complement to a complete cancer treatment plan.

One of the most remarkable uses of *Morinda citrifolia* is its use in the treatment of skin conditions. Noni juice can be applied directly to skin conditions, including minor burns, poison ivy, sunburns, skin infections, and a variety of rashes with remarkable results.

You will be hearing more and more about the amazing Noni plant as science investigates its uses and people around the world benefit from its many applications. I urge you to include this natural gift in your health improvement plan today. (See resources for information on how to get fresh Noni juice.)

10

POINTERS FOR A SUCCESSFUL EXERCISE PROGRAM

Today's world is full of modern conveniences, most of which are beneficial to mankind. Just a few years ago, we humans worked at hard physical labor all day just to feed ourselves. Today, a typical American meets this goal with an hour or two of sedentary office work. Work has become more mental and less physical. Someone else grows our food on a huge commercial farm, and then, far too often, a restaurant prepares the commercially grown food. Cars, trains, and planes carry us from place to place so that

IF YOU DON'T THINK IT IS A PRIVILEGE TO EXERCISE, HAVE A TALK WITH SOMEONE CONFINED TO A WHEELCHAIR.

we never break a sweat. We choose to ride the elevator or escalator, even if it takes longer to reach the next floor. All of these factors and more contribute to the growing epidemic of obesity and the diseases caused by a lack of exercise.

It has long been understood that exercise is good for the body. Both science and common sense tell us this. Yet America is abandoning the practice of habitual exercise. No medication, vitamin, or supplement can make up for this unfortunate trend. Exercise increases metabolism and activates immune response. It lowers blood pressure and blood sugar. Exercise helps keep bones, muscles, and hearts strong and efficient. Exercise also lifts moods and relieves pain. The benefits of even limited exercise are beyond doubt. To help initiate a pattern of long-term, frequent exercise, consider the following pointers as you undertake your exercise program.

Rx

RECOMMENDATIONS FOR A SUCCESSFUL EXERCISE PROGRAM

1. It is not necessary to run marathons to benefit from exercise.

2. You receive a health benefit from just twenty minutes of brisk walking four times a week. Do more if you

wish, but do at least this much. If your health has deteriorated to the point walking across the room is all you can exercise; do so at every opportunity. With time and effort most will see an improvement in exercise tolerance.

3. Purchase the best athletic shoes you can afford and replace them at least every six months.

4. If you run more than three to four miles per day six days per week for prolonged periods you will inevitably damage the weight-bearing joints. Competitive distance runners should slowly increase the distance run, timing the training to peak at the time of competition. After competition, the runner should follow with short distances and rest.

5. Short bursts of exercise throughout the day are almost as beneficial as prolonged periods of exercise. Take the stairs instead of the escalator. It all counts.

6. If you exercise in the morning, you are more likely to continue your habit of exercise in the future.

7. If you have several exercise options, you are more likely to continue to exercise.

8. Do something you enjoy for exercise. I enjoy gardening, and my wife, Cindy, enjoys riding horses. If you would rather chase a ball around than walk, do so with golf or basketball.

9. Attaining muscle symmetry, strength, and flexibility is the best way to prevent athletic injuries. A muscle that has a temperature of 101 degrees is most supple and willing to stretch. Warm up your muscles with a brisk walk or jog until you break a sweat, then stretch. Do not overwork one side of the body, as it is possible to do when you play only tennis for exercise. Create a balanced program for body symmetry.

10. Weight lifting is an excellent exercise option. By making more repetitions with less weight, weight lifting becomes an aerobic exercise.

11. If you lift weights in your exercise program, do not focus on the same muscle groups on successive days. Instead, work the chest and back muscles on Monday, Tuesday do aerobics, on Wednesday work the leg muscles, on Thursday do aerobics again, and on Friday work the arm muscles.

12. To complement your weight-lifting program, prior to lifting take a brisk walk or jog for a few minutes to

warm up your muscles. After lifting weights, stretch your warm muscles. Incorporating warm-ups and cool-down stretching helps to prevent athletic injuries.

13. It is not necessary to consume huge amounts of protein supplements to add bulk to your muscles. A healthy intestinal tract and kidneys can process up to one pound of pure protein a day without danger if adequate water is consumed. Meat, fish, and poultry are about 25 percent protein.

14. Contrary to popular belief, exercise is not a rapid way to lose weight. In fact, the average person must walk for ten hours at 3.5 miles per hour to lose just one pound of fat. This equals thirty-five miles of walking. This is based on the fact that one pound of fat represents 3,500 calories of stored energy. If we walk at a rate of 3.5 miles per hour we burn 350 calories an hour, requiring ten hours of walking to lose one pound of fat. Any weight loss above this amount is water loss. Understand that exercise reduces appetite and has a remarkable ability to normalize the desire for nutritional foods. Exercise also increases the metabolic rate for up to twenty-four hours after completion so that we burn more calories after exercise, even while we sleep.

15. Do not allow the weather to dictate if you exercise. Have indoor and outdoor options available. A successful pattern of exercise should not be brought to a halt by a cold front.

16. Eat a modest meal prior to exercise. The old adage of no food prior to a swim is groundless. The best schedule is breakfast first, then a workout.

17. If I could have only one form of exercise it would be a brisk walk in a beautiful park at sunrise. What a great way to start the day!

Richard L. Becker, .D.O.

Although we are all unique, my life experience has taught me that the things we have in common far exceed those which distinguish us from each other.

Fundamental human needs have not changed for thousands of years. We all need proper nourishment, water, exercise, rest, love, and spiritual fulfillment. The signs and symptoms of the body's failings vary greatly and have, in many cases, been falsely labeled as symptoms of a disease; in reality, they are warnings that our basic human needs are simply not being met. Your treatment for a health condition might be a little different from the next person's, but the fundamental needs of life must be met in order for your treatment program to succeed. You now have a foundation for the next step in healing, the application of remedies specifically tailored for your failing health syndrome.

PART II

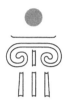

Have you ever had a long-term health problem? Perhaps the condition has progressed slowly and in spite of minor self-imposed adjustments the problem persists. You seek advice from a medical professional hoping for relief, only to be disappointed by the doctor's impatience and hurried manner.

In today's world of managed health care and HMO insurance plans, time-honored remedies and medical wisdom are all too frequently left out of the plan for wellness in the interest of time and money. It was once a common practice of family doctors to sit for a time with their patients and share their wisdom and experience in the healing arts.

The following section deals with a few of the most common chronic problems we suffer from and their time-honored holistic remedies. One reason these problems are so common and difficult to treat is that antidote medications do not cure these conditions. Many are forced to go from doctor to doctor, hoping the next one has the magic bullet to relieve their suffering, only to be disappointed. The answer to the problem is not an antidote but a complete holistic treatment method, a method that promotes healing from within.

The recommendations that follow can be used by virtually anyone. As a rule, they do not interact with medications and will not interfere with your doctor's treatment plan. (There are a few exceptions, which are clearly noted in the text.) It would be a good idea to share what you are doing with your doctor and pharmacist. Obviously, a book cannot replace your doctor, nor can it diagnose disease, but it can help you become more involved with your plan for wellness.

I urge you to read through the various conditions and their treatment, even if you do not suffer from them. Consider their commonality. This unity is the essence of the holistic approach to the treatment of disease. The astute reader will note early on the importance of a healthy intestinal tract and the principles used to correct a dysfunctional one.

If you gain but one thing from reading this book, I hope it is realizing that what you do on a daily basis, what you eat and drink, what medications you take, and how you approach your daily life challenges have a profound effect on your future health.

11

ARTHRITIS: JOINT AND SPINE PAIN

Joint and spine pain are among the most common reasons people seek the help of heath care professionals today. The causes of spine and joint pain are many, but the most common reasons include osteoarthritis, spinal stenosis, degenerative disc disease, ruptured discs, sprains and strains of the neck and back, and

A DOCTOR OR THERAPIST SKILLED IN THE USE OF THE THERAPEUTIC HAND IS A FRIEND TO KEEP FOR LIFE.

asymmetry of the musculoskeletal system. When finely tuned, healthy joints can help you achieve great things, but when out of order they can cause great suffering and disability.

Osteoarthritis is very common and frequently complicates the other painful conditions listed above. Osteoarthritis can be initiated by an injury, or it can be the result of years of wear and tear and poor dietary habits. The knees, hips, and spine are the joints most often affected, but this painful condition can afflict any joint. The medical community considers osteoarthritis incurable and is quick to prescribe anti-inflammatory medication to relieve the pain. These medications help in controlling the symptoms but do nothing to correct the underlying disorder and may cause serious side effects while in some instances actually delay healing.

Bones and joints are living tissues capable of healing. If the joints and spine are in mechanical balance and have the nutrients they need, they can heal.

The human organism is the most complex structure ever created. A special symmetry of structure is required for it to work efficiently. If the spine is not in the proper balance, stress points occur, which can greatly accelerate the degenerative processes associated with aging.

Our increasingly sedentary life style denies the spine the necessary strengthening motions to maintain vital health. As we age, our bodies lose their youthful flexibility, particularly if we sit or are inactive for prolonged periods of time in daily routines. If there is a history of an athletic or motor vehicle injury, followed by extended periods of inactivity, the body has been denied the corrective effects of exercise. If this scenario is combined with nutritional deficiencies, years of unnecessary pain and dysfunction from spinal conditions and osteoarthritis may result.

Years may pass from the time of initial injury to the development of osteoarthritis that can be demonstrated on an X ray. Many patients experience pain in this interim phase, sometimes before the doctor can see the cause of the pain. For optimal results, this is the time to intervene with a complete healing program, including hands-on therapy from your osteopath, chiropractor, or physical therapist to help restore the critical spine and joint balance needed for vital health. The program should also include a gentle exercise regimen to improve blood flow and strengthen the spine or injured joints, along with the essential vitamins, minerals, and supplements required for full healing.

If we do not address the healing needs of the injured area, chronic pain is inevitable. When we suffer in pain for extended periods of time, bad things happen. Sleep is disturbed. Depression sets in. Movement causes pain, so we exercise less and become weaker still. Stress of chronic pain can inhibit the immune system and cause hypertension. The sense of pleasant anticipation of future events or favorable outcomes is diminished, and each day becomes an endurance test. In a failing attempt to soothe and comfort, diet may become more of a means of pleasure than nourishment, and weight gain often results.

In an attempt to relieve pain, medications are often justifiably prescribed. Unfortunately, the medications used to control pain and inflammation of the spine and joints can cause intestinal inflammation, constipation, or diarrhea, resulting in an intestinal tract where the absorption of nutrients and elimination of wastes has been handicapped. Stress can become intense, causing a ripple effect of events that greatly affects the body's ability to heal and opens the door to many diseases.

An often overlooked tool in the management of osteoarthritis and painful spinal and joint conditions is osteopathic manipulative therapy. The osteopathic profession has received unjust criticism for not scientifically proving the merit of hands-on, manipulative therapy. Yet these studies have been done. Spinal manipulation lessens the need for medication and shortens the time patients perceive pain from their injuries. Spinal manipulation and hands-on therapy are among our most ancient forms of healing. There are writings dating back to the time of Hippocrates that refer to the virtue of the skilled therapeutic hand. For my allopathic friends, I would add that the scientific method begins with observation. It has been my observation, along with thousands of osteopaths, that manipulation is of great value when provided by experienced hands. Some things are intuitive and obvious. It is medication that requires double-blind studies and statistical evaluation, for the possible side effects of these treatments may be quite dangerous.

Osteopathic manipulative therapy's corrective benefits can best be understood by exploring the sequence of events initiated by a joint or spinal injury. The injury may seem mild and cause only minimal pain initially, but invariably a painful inflammatory response will occur. This, in turn, creates involuntary guarding and stiffness of the injured area. Anyone who has sprained an ankle knows how quickly the ankle becomes swollen and stiff. The supporting connective tissues of the ankle contract in order to protect the area. This guarding and stiffness will continue for several weeks and in some cases last well past the time required to heal the joint. After the initial period of healing, the patient then must actively restore the motion of the ankle with gentle stretching and strengthening exercises, or a state of chronic pain and instability of the ankle may result. But when the complicated spine, with dozens of joints and capable of almost infinite variations of motion, is injured, this pattern of guarding and stiffness may last for years, creating abnormal spinal and muscular stress points, which cause pain and greatly accelerate the body's normal degenerative process. Osteopathic manipulative therapy simply helps the injured joint or spine return to its full range of pain-free motion. If joint and spine motion is not restored over time, an X ray will show a reason for pain—osteoarthritis—but by this time a full return to health is unlikely.

I HAVE NEVER MET A PERSON WHO HAS OVERCOME DISABLING SPINE PAIN, WHO DID NOT INCLUDE PHYSICAL CONDITIONING ON THE ROAD TO RECOVERY.

It has also been my experience that another key to stopping this syndrome of chronic joint pain (before it becomes a permanent companion) is to diligently seek other causes that perpetuate the guarding and splinting of the spine or injured joint.

An anatomically short leg is a major perpetuator of spinal, joint, and muscle pain. In such cases, the spine is resting on a base that isn't level, and painful curves will have been created to compensate. The difference in leg lengths that can cause and perpetuate pain may be as little as one-fourth of an inch. It is not hard to imagine that one extremity could grow a little longer than the other, and if you have had a broken leg at any time in your life the likelihood of such a disproportion is even greater.

Poor posture, with an associated imbalance of muscle strength, is another perpetrator of spine pain. Repetitive imbalanced one-way motion such as that which occurs in a golf swing or in assembly-line work has caused pain for many people. Carrying a young child on the hip while doing household chores is another source of spine pain. The simple practice of standing up, stretching, and walking around every twenty to thirty minutes while at work goes a long way toward relieving such pain, especially when it is combined with a sensible exercise program. The full list of factors that can perpetuate such pain is long, but the concept is not complex. With dedication the cause can usually be found and corrective measures instituted.

After evaluating and determining the perpetuating factors, a program of rehabilitation must be established. This too is not complicated. Simply put, the patient must become strong and active again. Physical therapists can help you restore strength and mobility without reinjury.

IF HOT WATER AND A JOLT OF ELECTRICITY TRULY MADE BACK PAIN BETTER, PLUMBERS AND ELECTRICIANS WOULD BE TREATING SPINAL INJURY PATIENTS.

In severe cases, it is not unusual for a full response to treatment to take up to eighteen months. Injury to bone and tough connective tissues takes longer to heal than soft-tissue injuries, such as cuts and abrasions. Motion and strength are generally restored first, followed by an eventual reduction of pain.

Rest assured that pain relief will come when all the above factors—a search for perpetuating factors, physical therapy and conditioning, osteopathic manipulative therapy, and a complete nutritional program—are holistically combined.

Rx

RECOMMENDATIONS FOR ARTHRITIS: SPINE, AND JOINT PAIN

1. If you have gained weight, have any coexisting fungal infection, such as fungal toenails or recurrent yeast infections, or have taken steroids (cortisone, prednisone, dexamethasone, epidural steroid injection etc.), hormone replacement therapy, oral birth control pills, multiple rounds of antibiotics, or have taken antibiotics for prolonged periods of time at any time in your life, for best results include the HEALING DIET in your joint relief plan. If you do not require the HEALING DIET, you will attain the best results by stopping all dairy products except yogurt, cream, sour cream, cottage cheese, and butter, all carbonated beverages, all the nightshade plant foods (tomatoes, potatoes, eggplants, peppers, and tobacco) and by following the DIET FOR THE REST OF YOUR LIFE.

2. If you have any co-existing health condition with spinal or joint pain institute proper management principles for that condition. Many chronic pain patients find their pain mysteriously improves when other health conditions are brought under control.

3. If you have diabetes refer to the chapter dedicated to diabetes and include the following supplements in your plan for wellness.

    a. Alpha lipoic acid: 300-900 mg daily. (CAUTION: may lower blood sugar.)

    b. Chromium picolinate: 400-800 mcg daily. (CAUTION: may lower blood sugar.)

4. If you are in pain and have a history of thyroid problems or have a low body temperature refer to Dr. E. Denis Wilson's book, Wilson's Temperature Syndrome: A Reversible Low Temperature Problem. The book can be read online for free at www.wtsmed.com

5. Consult your osteopath or chiropractor for hands-on manipulative therapy and to determine if physical therapy may be of help.

6. Start a gentle exercise program that will not aggravate your painful joints. Swimming, bicycling, and walking in good, supportive athletic shoes will help restore your strength and blood circulation without causing further damage to your joints. Seek the help of your physical therapist to direct your exercise program. Ask your physical therapist for a home based stretching and flexibility program. Stretching is most effective after exercise while your muscles are warm.

7. Include the sulphur-rich foods in your diet. Eggs, onion, and garlic help your bones and connective tissues heal. Eat tart red cherries frequently or take a cherry fruit extract supplement, as cherries contain a natural pain-relieving substance. Include the spices turmeric, ginger, rosemary and royal jelly in your diet as they calm inflammation.

8. If your doctor has prescribed a nonsteroidal anti-inflammatory drug such as ibuprofen to control your pain, consider taking deglycyrrhizinated licorice (DGL). This form of licorice has been shown to help prevent the intestinal irritation commonly caused by these arthritis agents, without raising your blood pressure as nontreated licorice can do. A typical dose is DGL 380 mg 1–4 capsules prior to meals, 3 times daily.

9. Calcium: 1,000–2,000 mg daily.

10. Magnesium: 500–1,000 mg daily.

11. Sea kelp: 1–2 grams daily for trace minerals including boron, selenium, manganese, and copper.

12. B-Complex: 50 mg 3 times daily.

13. Vitamin C: 1–3 grams daily.

14. Essential Amino Acid supplement: 2 grams daily.

15. Vitamin E: 400 I.U. daily.

16. High potency multiple vitamin, mineral an amino acid powder: 1 tbs daily may be used in place of numbers 9-15.

17. Glucosamine sulfate: 300 mg up to 5 tablets daily.

18. Chondroitin sulfate: 200 mg up to 5 tablets daily.

19. Methylsulfonylmethane (MSM): 300 mg up to 5 tablets daily.

20. Counter irritant spray containing menthol or hot

pepper extract (capsaicin): spray on affected area as needed for quick pain relief.

21. Noni juice: 1–6 oz daily. For best pain relief take small amounts several times throughout the day and before bedtime.

22. Probiotics with fructo-oligosaccharides: 1-2 capsules daily for 3–6 months then 1-2 capsules per week thereafter and whenever you may require antibiotic treatment in the future.

23. Glucomannan fiber: 575 mg 3-9 capsules daily with a large glass of water. This soluble fiber source is remarkably well tolerated. Psyllium: 1 tbs in water daily is another fiber option.

24. Beta glucan: 10 mg 1 or 2 daily. For best results, take with Noni juice on an empty stomach.

25. Grape seed-extracted oligomeric proanthocyanidins (OPC) with at least 95% active component purity: 100–200 mg daily.

26. Fish or flaxseed oil with borage seed oil: 3–5 grams of each daily.

27. If your condition is giving you the "blues," add:

a. St. Johns Wort: 300 mg, 1–3 capsules daily. (DO NOT TAKE ST. JOHNS WORT WITH ANY ANTIDEPRESSANT MEDICATION.)

b. SAMe: 400 mg 1 tablet twice daily. (DO NOT TAKE SAMe WITH ANY ANTIDEPRESSANT MEDICATION)

Richard L. Becker, .D.O.

12

AUTOIMMUNE DISEASES

The medical literature describes and classifies some seventy different types of diseases as the autoimmune diseases. These diseases vary in presentation but have in common the phenomena of the immune system mistakenly attacking various body parts as though they were an infectious agent or a foreign object. In short, your immune system is no longer your friend but your worst enemy. Rheumatoid arthritis, insulin-dependent diabetes, sarcoidosis, systemic lupus erythematosus, and Graves' disease are but a few examples of these increasingly prevalent disorders.

TODAY'S MEDICAL STANDARD OF CARE IS TOMORROW'S BAD MEDICINE.

This same medical literature describes in tedious detail how the misdirected immune system can slowly incapacitate the patient, creating a life of endless debilitation. It does not tell us the true cause or how to cure the condition. In no other area of the treatment of human suffering is the difference between allopathic medicine and holistic medicine so glaring. The allopath attempts to suppress immunity with steroids and immune-modulating antidotes, while the holist attempts to normalize and heal with a balance of nature's corrective nutrients and plant extracts.

The successful treatment of these diseases, with any method, requires early intervention. There is a point of no return in which our only remedy is relief of pain. If the patient is willing and has but a small reserve of strength, there is still hope for a better day.

Do not think for a minute that modern science knows all there is to know. The workings of the human body are far more complicated than any machine man has ever devised. I do not pretend to have all the answers to the autoimmune diseases, but I can tell you what I have seen. If the damage to the organs involved is not too great, these diseases can be slowed and in many cases stopped.

It is only fair to call this correction a state of remission and not a cure, just as we call a good therapeutic response in cancer a remission. The propensity to develop an autoimmune disease is present in some form in all of us. These conditions certainly run in families, yet not all family members develop the disease. There is hope for you. But you must become involved in your treatment course, and you must be willing to make dramatic changes in your lifestyle.

Many of the people who suffer from the autoimmune diseases have several features in common. They are as follows:

1. Female gender. Not just because of the two X chromosomes but also because of the added burden of reproduction and the hormonal and nutritional stresses it creates.

2. Multiple antibiotic courses. Many have taken fifty or more rounds of antibiotics or have been on antibiotics for prolonged periods of time, such as the treatment of acne with tetracycline for a two-year period.

3. Steroid use. Any of the many forms of steroids may have been used, such as prescription allergy nasal sprays, oral birth control pills, prednisone,

dexamethasone, methylprednisolone, estrogen hormone replacement therapy, and others. Many of the autoimmune disease patients have used these steroid preparations for another seemingly unrelated condition many years in the past.

4. The combination of antibiotics with steroids seems to be a synergistic risk.

5. Continued allergies well into adulthood.

6. Chronic intestinal conditions such as chronic diarrhea, irritable bowel syndrome, or chronic constipation.

7. High-sugar diet. Please understand that just one serving per day of a sugared food must be considered a high-sugar diet.

8. Recurrent or chronic fungal infections such as fungal toenails, jock itch, ringworm, recurrent vaginal yeast infections, or tinea versicolor.

9. Multiple doctor interventions and medication use. The autoimmune patient typically has a prolonged period of failing health that requires multiple doctor evaluations and remedies before the pattern of the autoimmune disease emerges.

10. Some medications alone can cause an autoimmune disease state.

If these factors are present in your history but you have not been diagnosed with an autoimmune disease, consider this a warning. Implementation of the following recommendations may prevent considerable misery in your life. If you have these risk factors and have been diagnosed with an autoimmune disease, there is a good chance that these measures will greatly help you regain your health and vitality. Please be aware that in general these recommendations will not go against what your doctor has prescribed for you. In fact you may find them complementary to your doctor's treatment, making the medications more effective. It is always in your best interest to share what you're doing with your doctor so that he or she may help you adapt your healing program to your special needs.

YOU MAY HAVE INHERITED A TENDENCY FOR DISEASE, BUT YOU HAVE ALSO INHERITED THE ABILITY TO HEAL.

Rx _____

RECOMMENDATIONS FOR AUTOIMMUNE DISEASES

1. Follow the HEALING DIET for as long as it takes. Be prepared for a significant healing crisis. Refer

to Chapter 7, which is dedicated to this topic. Many people find that as long as they are on the HEALING DIET they do well, so they elect to remain on their version of the HEALING DIET for life. I recommend that you attempt to progress through the TRANSITIONAL DIET to the DIET FOR THE REST OF YOUR LIFE as tolerated.

2. Ladies: If PMS or menopause symptoms accompanies you're autoimmune condition refer to Chapter 19 MENOPAUSE MANAGEMENT THE NATURAL WAY and include the recommendations in your treatment plan as hormonal swings can greatly aggravate your condition.

3. If you have any co-existing health condition with your autoimmune disorder institute proper management principles. Autoimmune diseases are complex, illusive and often misdiagnosed. By controlling any other co-existing health condition you may initiate a spontaneous remission of your autoimmune disease.

4. If you're autoimmune condition involves the thyroid gland or you have a low body temperature refer to Dr. E. Denis Wilson's book, Wilson's Temperature Syndrome: A Reversible Low Temperature Problem. The book can be read online for free at www.wtsmed.com.

5. Drink more water: 1/2 oz filtered water per pound of body weight daily. Chronic dehydration has a profound effect on the immune system and its occurrence may mimic autoimmune disease.

6. High potency multiple vitamin, mineral and amino acid powder: 1 tbs daily.

7. Beta glucan: 10 mg 1 or 2 times daily to help normalize immune function.

8. Noni juice: 2–4 oz daily.

9. Glucomannan fiber: 575 mg 3-9 capsules daily with a large glass of water. This soluble fiber source is remarkably well tolerated. Psyllium: 1 tbs in water daily is another fiber option. Avoid fiber agents that contain starch or sugar while on the HEALING DIET.

10. Probiotics with fructo-oligosaccharides: 1-2 capsules daily for 3–6 months then 1-2 capsules per week thereafter and whenever you may require antibiotic treatment in the future.

11. Fish oil or flaxseed oil with borage seed oil: 2–4 grams of each daily.

12. Grape seed-extracted oligomeric proanthocyanidins (OPC) with at least 95% active component purity: 200 mg daily.

13. Milk thistle extract (Silybum marianum) standardized to deliver 70–80% silymarin: 200 mg 3 times daily.

14. Coenzyme Q10/L-carnitine: 30 mg/250 mg 1 or 2 capsules daily.

15. Quercetin: 500 mg daily.

16. Glucosamine sulfate: 300 mg up to 5 times daily.

17. Chondroitin sulfate: 200 mg up to 5 times daily.

18. Methylsulfonylmethane (MSM): 300 mg up to 5 times daily.

19. Juice with fresh carrots and any other vegetables or fruits allowed on the HEALING DIET, 6-12 oz daily.

20. The following have antiyeast and antifungal properties. Many find help by cycling through each supplement to suppress intestinal yeast growth. You may also combine these agents if needed. If you are intolerant of any, discontinue its use and advance to

the next agent. If you find one agent that is particularly helpful, continue the agent for as long as necessary.

a. Pau d'arco: 500 mg 1–4 capsules twice daily, days 1–30

b. Caprylic acid: 500 mg 1–4 capsules twice daily, days 31–60

c. Oil of oregano: 5–10 drops or 1-2 gel caps once or twice daily, days 61–90·

d. Olive leaf: 100 mg 1–2 capsules daily, days 91–120

e. Garlic: 3–5 grams daily, days 121–150

f. Unpasteurized apple cider vinegar: 1 tsp in 8 oz water, once or twice daily, days 151–180.

21. Emphasize onions, garlic, and eggs in your diet as these foods contain sulfur rich amino acids.

22. Include the spices turmeric, ginger, rosemary, oregano leaf and royal jelly in your diet or as a supplement as they calm inflammation.

23. Stop all dairy products except cream, sour cream, yogurt, kefir and butter.

24. Limit your exposure to chemicals (pesticides, etc.) and excessive sunlight.

25. Eliminate the nightshade family of plants (eggplant, peppers, tomatoes, and potatoes) from your diet, as they are known to aggravate autoimmune disorders.

Richard L. Becker, .D.O.

13

CANCER

I cannot think of any three words that strike more fear in a person than, "You have cancer." Over 1.6 million Americans are told these same words every year. And 1.6 million families are forever changed.

There are four million Americans currently being treated for cancer. As a nation, we spend in over all costs, $200 billion annually in an ever-too-frequent failing attempt to save these lives.

The Universal Almanac reports that in 1900 only 3 percent of us died from

THE GREATEST GIFT A DOCTOR CAN GIVE A PATIENT IS THE ABILITY TO FUNCTION IN GOOD HEALTH INDEPENDENT OF A DOCTOR.

cancer. Today the figure is 25 percent. Certainly some of the deaths in 1900 were misdiagnosed, but let me assure you that the look of a patient dying of cancer is unmistakable. Early detection of this disease is a challenge and is far more difficult than recognizing its depredations. Space-age technology allows us to see the cancer tumor while it is still quite small. Even when a cancer is small in size, it may have been present too long for some patients to find a cure.

It is not hard to understand why cancer deaths have increased. The world is a polluted place, and more people are living longer than ever. The standard American diet is refined and depleted of nutrients. Our lives are but one stressful moment after another. According to the Harvard University School of Health, 65 percent of all cancers are due to unhealthy lifestyle practices. This may explain why we have more cancer, but it does not explain why we have done so poorly in curing the disease.

We must do better than this; we owe it to the world and to ourselves.

It is the opinion of many researchers today that chemotherapy has reached its maximum effectiveness. If it gets any stronger, we will kill patients before we rid their bodies of cancer. To win this battle, we must come to understand the fundamental cause of cancer in all its forms and correct the aberration before the disease sets in. We must address the fact that 40 percent of all cancer deaths are actually due to starvation and malnutrition, not the cancer. In order to maximize cure rates, we must treat the malnutrition and maximize the patient's immune response, while decreasing the tumor burden through selective agents designed to harm only the cancer and not the patient.

I do, however, want you to have hope, for there have been great advances in recent years, and the goal of effective cancer treatment is slowly being achieved. Thousands are alive today because they combined, when appropriate, the best modern pharmaceutical chemotherapy agents, debulking surgery, radiation, and immune-boosting extracts of nature's foods, along with scientifically proven dietary measures.

In our bodies, the battle with cancer goes on daily. It is happening within you, even while you are reading this book. It is thought the average healthy eighty-year-old has already

THE USE OF MEDICATION IS ALWAYS A COMPROMISE, BUT A COMPROMISE THAT MAY SAVE YOUR LIFE.

fought off cancer six times. To cure more cancer patients, we must know why this normally successful effort begins to fail. In some victims it is obvious. Their lifestyles contributed heavily to their failure. Yet others did the same harmful things and won the battle with cancer, never succumbing. Obviously, cancer is complicated, and the learning curve is steep and jagged. This is no place for the novice climber who has just heard those dreaded words: "You have cancer."

What would you do? Trust a stranger with your life? Hope that stranger will have complete knowledge of what to do and do it right?

I cannot answer this for you, but I can tell you what I did when I heard those dreaded words. I found the first step to healing was acceptance of the disease. It did not come immediately. It took a while. I fought with denial for a long time, almost too long. Every fiber of my being wanted to run, run from those words, "You have cancer." If it were not for my wife and family, I probably would have kept running. But they needed me, all of me, for a very long time. At first, I fought for them. But fighting did not cure the disease. I had to surrender. Just as you surrender to God when you finally realize you cannot do it alone, you must surrender your will to healing.

Next, I had to realize my humanity. We all die. The question is when. If this is the end, you must accept what you cannot change. No one has the tools or energy to change what you yourself cannot.

These two steps put my mind at ease. You must take these two steps as well. Understand it is not only up to you.

The next step was accepting the help offered, as you will need to do. Your family loves you, and they want to show you how much you mean to them with their nurturing. Let them. They need to show their love as much as you need their love.

After your family and soul are unified, seek professional help and include your family doctor, oncologist, and a nutritionist experienced in the treatment of cancer. You cannot leave the entire burden to them. You must read and learn all you can about the nutritional methods used today to complement cancer treatment. If you are too weak to do so, your loved ones will assist you in this endeavor.

I urge you not to pursue unproven modalities in distant places. There are many charlatans waiting to profit from your ignorance and desperation. However, accept legitimate options supported by studies from any country, as the United States is not necessarily at the forefront in all scientific endeavors. The world is now a small place. The serious student of cancer treatment accepts valid information from any legitimate source.

The current state of the art in cancer treatment is, when appropriate, to decrease the gross mass of the tumors by surgery, radiation, and chemotherapy, to maximize the patient's immune potential and nutritional status, and to provide social and spiritual support.

We have no means at the current time to detect cancer at the cellular level. If a tumor is visible on X rays and scans, there is a high degree of probability of an undetected spread of the disease, which may be hiding in very small nests of metastatic tumor growth. This phenomenon makes it imperative to treat the cancer in some form for the life of the patient. It is shortsighted to believe cancer will never return in this setting.

Once you have consulted with your panel of cancer treatment experts and the treatment course has been decided, expect a difficult road. Many of the treatments are toxic and challenging to endure. If your cancer can be cut out, it should be, but the treatment is not over. You must support your healing process so that the disease does not come back, and you will need to do this for the rest of your life. If your course of treatment includes chemotherapy, expect some dramatic changes, which no advice can prepare you for. Some patients virtually breeze through chemotherapy, while others become very sick. Chemotherapy affects all cells that reproduce quickly, including those of the hair follicles, bone marrow, and digestive tract, causing your hair to fall out, anemia, and nausea with vomiting. Perhaps the most profound effect is on the brain and how it makes you feel. Sleep patterns can be dramatically affected; depression may set in, leaving you feeling poorly equipped to carry on. This is a stage we must simply endure. There are medications to help alleviate the adverse reactions. Mostly what is needed is endurance. This is where nutritional measures play a major role. They will help support your ability to endure until your system takes the upper hand and begins to heal.

If all goes well and the day comes when your oncologist tells you, "You're in remission," expect the next major hurdle in your path. This stage is perplexing. You have now heard the best news you could ever hear, yet you do not know if you can go on. You do not feel cured. You are tired; you ache all over; you are depressed and do not know why your life has been spared when so many other lives have been lost. This stage of cancer healing was the most difficult for me and for many others who are now cancer survivors. For many it is too much to endure alone. You must find a reason to go on. God did not spare your life for nothing. Someone somewhere needs you. You may not know who. It is now your job to find out. When Job endured all that any human could endure, his reward was to return to work. He did not win the lottery, did he? He returned to what we humans do so proficiently when

vitally healthy—work. Find the job you survived cancer to do.
Perhaps your hospital needs a volunteer. Or your neighbor was
just diagnosed with cancer, and your counsel would be of help.
Do not wait for this purpose to come to you. Seek it out!

Once you have found your reason for healing, learn to love
your new body, for it has changed. Respect the changes;
consider them badges of honor. Eat every meal with your
good health in mind. Support your nutrition with the best
supplements you can afford. And thank God daily for every
rose on your path and every sunset on the horizon.

Rx

COMPLEMENTS TO YOUR CANCER TREATMENT

1. The first priority of cancer treatment is the relief of
   suffering and the maintenance of dignity.

2. There is hope. Believe it. Live it.

3. Your spirit must be at
   peace to heal.

   A GOOD ATTITUDE WILL HELP YOU THROUGH MOST ANYTHING.

4. Explore your options. If
   there is any doubt, seek a second opinion. Formulate
   a plan, then stick to it.

5. Formulate and follow a diet that is absolutely free of white sugar and low in starches and carbohydrates. The HEALING DIET is an appropriate choice.

6. Ninety percent of all cancers are due to environmental toxic overload. Avoid exposure to mold, pesticides, tobacco smoke, alcohol, powerful cleaning solutions, artificial food coloring agents, paints, etc. This stress must be relieved in order to succeed.

7. Lower the tumor burden with surgery, chemotherapy, and radiation as appropriate with the help of your oncologist.

8. Do not pointlessly pursue experimental toxic therapies to gratify you or your doctor's need to do something.

9. If you become too weak to prepare and consume the HEALING DIET, consider IMMUNE POWER liquid meal replacement supplement: to order call 888-741-LIFE.

10. Assure that your immune system has all it needs to heal you. Vitamins alone will not cure your cancer! But if you have a deficiency of any essential dietary element, your efforts will be futile. Take high-quality, absorbable vitamins, minerals, and amino acid supplements. A high potency multiple vitamin,

mineral and amino acid powder (1 tbs daily) is an appropriate choice.

11. Supplement the essential fatty acids with flaxseed or fish oil with borage seed oil: 2-4 grams of each daily.

12. Drink juices daily made from fresh fruits and vegetables allowed on the HEALING DIET. (Recent studies show 6 oz. of pomegranate juice daily may stabilize PSA levels in patients with prostate cancer.)

13. Include a fiber supplement such as glucomannan or psyllium, dosage as tolerated to help detoxify the effects of cancer treatment and to promote regularity.

14. Probiotic with fructo-oligosaccharide: 1-2 tablets daily to maintain bowel flora.

15. Improve immune function with the following:

   a. Beta glucan: 10 mg, 1 capsule twice daily for the rest of your life. Beta glucans have been shown to protect the patient from the side effects of radiation therapy.

   b. Noni juice: 16 oz daily for 4 days, followed by 8 oz daily for 4 days, followed by 4 oz daily for the rest of your life.

c. IP-6: 800 mg, 2 capsules twice daily for the rest of your life.

d. Inositol: 220 mg, 2 capsules twice daily for the rest of your life.

e. Garlic: 3 grams daily.

f. Colostrum: 1 gram daily.

g. Echinacea purpurea: 80 mg daily.

h. Curcumin: 50 mg daily.

i. Algesic acid: 100 mg daily.

j. Cabbage extracted indole-3 carbinol: 200 mg daily.

16. Coenzyme Q10/L-carnitine: 30 mg/250 mg 2-4 gel caps daily. This supplement is critical for cardiovascular protection if you are taking chemotherapy.

17. Milk thistle extract (Silybum marianum) standardized to deliver 70–80% silymarin: 200 mg 1–3 times daily for liver support.

18. To prevent Candida and yeast overgrowth, include any two of the following:

    a. Caprylic acid: 500 mg 2 times daily

    b. Pau d'arco: 500 mg 2 times daily

    c. Oil of oregano: 2–6 drops in water twice daily

    d. Leaf of oregano: 100 mg twice daily

    e. Unpasteurized apple cider vinegar: 1 tsp in water twice daily

    f. Olive leaf extract: 100 mg 1–2 capsules twice daily.

19. Melatonin: 3–24 mg 1 hour prior to bed for sleep. Use the lowest dose possible to initiate sleep.

20. Gentle exercise as often as tolerated. If you can walk only across the room, do so as often as you can.

21. Include your osteopath, physical therapist, or chiropractor in your treatment plan if possible.

22. Take megadose vitamins only under the supervision of your doctor.

23. Enjoy a little sunshine on your face whenever possible as vitamin D is a potent cancer fighter.

24. Enjoy laughter on a daily basis. Choose a happy, funny movie instead of a drama or sad one.

25. Become active in the "Cancer Survivor Club" as soon as possible. Find a reason for your survival.

26. If you are doing all you can, yet not gaining ground, treat aggressively for a fungal condition. This will require prescriptive antifungal medication. There are many recorded cases of "cancer" remission when treated as a fungus.

Richard L. Becker, .D.O.

A HOSPITAL IS NO PLACE TO GET WELL.

14

DIABETES MELLITUS

Diabetes mellitus is a metabolic disorder that results in a condition of persistently elevated blood glucose (blood sugar). There are two basic types of diabetes, insulin-dependent diabetes, which has its onset early in life, and non-insulin-dependent diabetes, which begins relatively late in life. Type I diabetes accounts for 5 to 10 percent of all diabetes and

DESPITE THE BEST EFFORTS OF MODERN SCIENCE, NO MAN-MADE MEDICINE, HORMONE, OR MACHINE CAN MATCH WHAT NATURE CONTROLS THROUGH A HEALTHY SET OF ORGANS.

is an autoimmune disease. This is initiated by a viral infection, where damage has occurred to the pancreas, decreasing one's internal ability to control blood glucose. Type II diabetes is the result of resistance to the effects of insulin by several known mechanisms. Both types are capable of doing great damage and are associated with many coexisting diseases. Diabetes is the leading cause of preventable blindness, renal dialysis, and amputations. It is also a major risk factor for cardiovascular disease. There are twenty million Americans who have diabetes, and half of them do not know it. Diabetes is the sixth leading cause of death in the United States, and its occurrence is increasing.

The management of diabetes is best summarized by the saying, "an ounce of prevention is worth a pound of cure," as most of the complications can be prevented by good blood-glucose control and healthy lifestyle measures. The typical Type II diabetic is overweight and has a blood chromium level 40 percent lower than normal. The essential trace mineral chromium is normally found in "whole grain" and carbohydrate sources but is removed by the refinement process. This simple fact underscores the essence of nutrition-based disease and in diabetes, as with all diseases, any nutrient deficiency must be addressed for treatment success.

The following six principles must be accepted and applied by every diabetic in order to successfully manage their condition.

1. Diet is the most important treatment of diabetes. No matter how skilled your doctors are, or how advanced their medication is, if a proper diet is not in place the treatment will fail.

2. Patients must frequently check their blood glucose and record the readings. This diabetic diary provides both doctor and patient with critical information upon which therapeutic adjustments may be made. A reasonable blood glucose testing schedule would be just prior to breakfast (7 a.m.) and 3–4 hours after lunch (4 p.m.) or anytime you feel bad or exceptionally good.

3. Stress from any source, emotional or physical, raises blood glucose. Many diabetics can tell they are becoming ill from a cold or flu by a rise in blood glucose prior to feeling bad. Any sweet substance, including sugar, honey, molasses, or syrups, along with fruits and grain-derived foods raises blood glucose.

4. Exercise, insulin, diabetic medication, and a proper diet lower blood glucose. A low blood glucose would lessen the amount of the next diabetic medication dose or increase the calorie content of the next meal or snack or both.

5. Strive for an even flow of blood glucose readings. Try to avoid wide fluctuations of blood glucose.

6. You must become your own doctor if you are a diabetic. You must learn how to control your glucose by adjustments of medications, supplements, diet, and exercise. You cannot and should not see a doctor on a daily basis. You must know how to handle a low blood glucose attack or episodes of unusually high blood glucose. Obviously, there will be matters that require the attention of your physician, but the adjustments of daily living are up to you.

It is the wise and mature diabetic, Type I or II, who accepts these concepts early in the course of his disease. I cannot overemphasize their importance.

There is great concern among health care providers about the increasing incidence of Type II diabetes, and the reason is painfully obvious. We, as a nation, are overweight and eat an overly refined diet. Americans, on average, eat 155 pounds of sugar per year. We drink more soda than water. We walk no farther

THE LEAST AMOUNT OF MEDICATION TO DO THE JOB EFFECTIVELY IS ALWAYS THE BEST AMOUNT.

than from our homes to our cars and back again. Is it any wonder that diabetes is increasing?

I believe Type II diabetes can be prevented in most cases and reversed in others with healthy lifestyle measures. If you have been diagnosed with diabetes do not lose hope. There is help. The following measures will help to control your blood glucose and restore your sense of vitality.

Rx

RECOMMENDATIONS FOR THE DIABETIC

1. Type I insulin-dependent diabetics may use the DIET FOR THE REST OF YOUR LIFE or the American Diabetic Association (ADA) diet based on the carbohydrate exchange system. The ADA exchange diet equates 1 exchange for a measure of carbohydrate and is useful for learning the carbohydrate content of various foods. Even high-quality, nutritious foods such as watermelon may dramatically raise your blood sugar. The ADA diet, available from your doctor or registered dietician, helps you learn which foods will raise your blood sugar levels the most and which foods normalize blood glucose.

2. Type II diabetics who are overweight may follow the ADA exchange diet or the TRANSITIONAL DIET to lose weight slowly, at the overall rate of two to four pounds per month. With either approach, it is in your interest to replace some carbohydrate calories with calories from the essential fatty acid oils, olive, safflower, flaxseed, and fish oils. The normalization of your weight is imperative to your long-term well-being.

3. Incorporate the six fundamental principles listed above into your daily life and understand regular exercise is a critical component of the management of diabetes.

4. B-complex: 50 mg twice daily.

5. Vitamin C: 1 gram daily.

6. Vitamin A: 8,000 IU daily.

7. Vitamin E: 400 IU daily.

8. Calcium: 1 gram daily.

9. Magnesium: 500 mg daily.

10. Zinc: 15 mg daily.

11. Sea kelp: 1 gram daily.

12. High potency multiple vitamin, mineral and amino acid powder: 1 tbs daily with water may be substituted for numbers 4 through 11 above.

13. Chromium picolinate: 400–800 micrograms daily. Start with 200 micro-grams daily and check your blood sugar; advance up to 800 micro-grams daily. Many Type II diabetics achieve better blood glucose control with fewer medications when they supplement chromium.

14. Noni juice: 1-2 oz morning and evening.

15. Fish or flaxseed oil with borage seed oil: 2-4 grams of each daily.

16. Alpha-lipoic acid (ALA): 300-600 mg daily. ALA is a useful tool in the treatment and prevention of diabetic neuropathy. ALA is capable of lowering blood glucose.

17. Grape seed-extracted oligomeric proanthocyanidins (OPC) with at least 95% active component purity: 200 mg daily.

18. Beta glucan: 10 mg, 1 or 2 capsules daily

19. Coenzyme Q10/L-carnitine: 30 mg/250 mg 1-2 capsules daily.

20. Quercetin: 250 mg twice daily.

21. Glucomannan fiber: 575 mg 3-9 capsules daily with a large glass of water. This soluble fiber source is remarkably well tolerated and has been shown to lower blood glucose and cholesterol in diabetics. Psyllium: 1 tbs in water daily is another fiber option. Diabetics should avoid fiber agents that contain starch or sugar.

22. Probiotics with fructo-oligosaccharides: 1 tablet daily

23. Fenugreek and cinnamon teas are helpful remedies that lower blood glucose.

24. Make exercise a priority. A gentle daily walk has been shown to decrease the need for diabetic medications and improve blood glucose levels.

25. Take special care of your feet. Even a minor blister on a diabetic's foot can lead to amputation.

26. Lutein: 6 mg daily for eye health.

27. Zeaxanthin: .3 mg daily for eye health.

28. See your doctor at least annually for blood pressure checks and urine tests and a review of your diabetic diary. Include the doctor's laboratory data in your diabetic diary. Diabetes is a risk factor for many diseases, and early detection of these diseases is imperative. Bi-annual eye exams are recommended as diabetes is the leading cause of preventable blindness.

29. Oil of oregano: 5 drops in water or 1 gel cap daily for Candida treatment or prevention. Diabetics are highly susceptible to Candida, yeast, and fungal infections, making the patient overly prone to the fungal side effects of antibiotics, hormones, and steroids. If you require these types of medication, observe the recommendations listed in the chapter on fungal diseases.

30. The list of recommendations for the diabetic is long and may seem overwhelming. Keep in mind diabetes

is the leading cause of kidney failure, amputations, preventable blindness and it is a major risk factor for cardiovascular disease, the leading cause of death in America. An ounce of prevention is truly worth a pound of cure.

Richard L. Becker, .D.O.

ONE OF THE BEST FRIENDS A PERSON COULD HAVE IS A

CONCERNED AND INVOLVED PHARMACIST.

15

Gastroesophageal Reflux Disease and Peptic Ulcer Disease

Peptic ulcer disease (PUD) is a condition of ulceration or erosion of the upper intestinal lining. Any tissue that comes in contact with stomach acid may become ulcerated. Ulcers may occur from the lower esophagus to the upper part of the small intestine. The condition of peptic ulcers may be very painful, forcing the patient to seek immediate medical attention, or it may be subtle, requiring extensive testing to diagnose.

A HEALTHY LIVER AND INTESTINAL TRACT ARE FOUNDATIONS FOR A LONG, HEALTHY LIFE.

The great danger of peptic ulcer disease lies in its ability to erode into a blood vessel and cause bleeding, or penetrate the intestinal lining, creating a life-threatening condition.

Medical researchers have discovered that most peptic ulcers of the stomach and duodenum (first twelve inches of the small intestines) are the result of bacterial infection by Helicobacter pylori. Imagine the countless people with ulcers in the past who were told they could not handle the stresses of modern life and if they could only control themselves, their ulcers would go away. Proper antibiotics and anti-ulcer medication can eradicate these bacteria. Fortunately, since the development of these medications, the incidence of hemorrhage, surgery, and death from ulcers has sharply declined. But treating the ulcers only with antibiotics and acid-suppressive drugs does nothing to correct the underlying disorder, leaving the patient prone to recurrent intestinal infections and complications from the antibiotic and acid-suppression treatment.

While the incidence of peptic ulcer-related surgery and death has declined, the prevalence of gastroesophageal reflux disease (GERD) has dramatically increased. Commonly known as GERD or heartburn, GERD is a condition of stomach acid vaporizing or refluxing up the esophagus onto tissue unable to withstand the acidity. The bacterium Helicobacter pylori does not appear to have a role in GERD.

The same acid-suppressive medication used to treat peptic ulcers has been found to greatly reduce the pain and esophageal irritation of GERD. These medications are consistently among the best-selling drugs in America. But the suppression of stomach acid does nothing to correct the underlying disorder. The underlying disorder in peptic ulcers and GERD is but another manifestation of INTESTINAL DYSBIOSIS (See Chapter 4—THE BEGINNING TO THE END) and America's obvious trend toward obesity and malnourishment.

Intestinal dysbiosis is a condition of altered or abnormal microbial life forms in the intestines. The typical normal adult has approximately three pounds of bacteria, yeast, and assorted life forms in his or her intestinal tract. With the increasing use of antibiotics, steroids, hormones, and the propensity of Americans to eat huge amounts of sugar and refined foods, and to avoid raw foods, altered intestinal bacteria and yeast is inevitable.

According to the United States Department of Agriculture, at least half of all Americans consume a diet deficient in essential nutrients. This dietary deficiency leads to overeating of abnormal foods, as observed in the Pica syndrome model for abnormal food cravings (the eating of abnormal foods when iron deficient) and weight gain inevitably follows.

The typical heartburn sufferer has gained weight. A gain of just ten pounds is enough to aggravate and in some cases cause the condition of GERD. The patient may have taken various medications that alter the body's chemistry, such as hormone replacement therapy, antibiotics, antacids, and stomach acid-suppressive medications. Over time, the acid-suppressive medication interferes with digestion and may lead to further subclinical nutrient deficiencies that can greatly compromise health. Once the pattern of heartburn is established, it becomes a beast that perpetuates itself in overeating and continued daily medication for relief. For success in the treatment of GERD, the nutrient deficiencies and chemical imbalances created by these well-meaning medications must be corrected, and the added weight must be lost.

Due to the potential serious or even life-threatening nature of abdominal pain, you must seek the help of your physician. Once a proper diagnosis is made, you should include these measures in your recovery plan. The following recommendations are YOU ARE WHAT generally well tolerated, but it is always YOU EAT. a good idea to share your plan with your physician. Persistence pays off. Stay with this program. With time, those tummyaches will be a thing of the past.

Rx

RECOMMENDATIONS FOR GERD AND PEPTIC ULCER DISEASE

1. Exclude all aspirin, ibuprofen, naproxyn, and aspirin-like medications.

2. Eliminate all carbonated beverages and reduce your caffeine intake significantly.

3. Cut out all chocolate and mint foods.

4. Terminate all forms of tobacco use.

5. Be careful with onions, tomatoes, and citrus, as GERD and PUD may be exacerbated. Once you feel better, increase citrus and onions as tolerated because they are frequently consumed by the healthy and vital person.

6. Eat small, frequent meals and never skip breakfast.

7. Drink 1/2 oz filtered water per pound of body weight daily. Chronic dehydration alone can cause GERD and delay healing of an ulcer.

8. Do not lie down for 1 1/2 hours after eating.

9. Stop all milk products except those allowed on the HEALING DIET. Stop all sugar and refined foods.

10. Wear loose fitting comfortable clothing to avoid pressure on the abdomen.

11. If you have gained weight, taken oral birth control pills, hormone replacement therapy, steroid therapy, multiple antibiotics, or antibiotics for a prolonged period of time for any condition, follow the HEALING DIET for best results.

12. Juice with carrots, cabbage, and celery: 6-12 oz daily.

13. Vitamin A: 8,000 IU daily.

14. Vitamin C: 1 gram daily.

15. Vitamin E: 400 IU daily.

16. Zinc: 15 mg daily.

17. B-complex: 50 mg twice daily.

18. Calcium: 1 gram daily.

19. Magnesium: 500 mg daily.

20. Sea kelp: 1 gram daily.

21. Amino acid supplement: 2 grams daily.

22. High potency multiple vitamin, mineral and amino acid powder: 1 tbs daily in water may be used in place of numbers 13–21.

23. If you have a history of Helicobacter pylori, consider Mastic gum: 500 mg twice daily for two weeks. Mastic gum is derived from the pistachio tree and is native to the Greek islands. It has been shown to be effective and well tolerated for the treatment of Helicobacter pylori infections.

24. Beta glucan: 10 mg twice daily.

25. Noni juice: 1 oz prior to meals and bedtime until pain free, then 1–2 oz daily.

26. L-Glutamine: 500 mg 3 times daily.

27. Fish or flaxseed oil with borage seed oil: 2 grams of each daily.

28. Probiotics with fructo-oligosaccharides: 1-2 tablets on an empty stomach daily for 6 months, then 1-2 tablets taken once weekly thereafter.

29. Glucomannan fiber: 575 mg 4-6 capsules daily with a large glass of water. Psyllium: 1 tbs in water daily is another fiber option.

Richard L. Becker, .D.O.

PERSISTENCE PAYS OFF . . . .

YOU HAVE NO CHOICE BUT TO GET WELL.

16

WHY ARE AMERICANS
DYING OF HEART DISEASE?

During the 1960s, it became evident that increased numbers of Americans were dying from heart disease and stroke. The cost of this disease has been high, both in suffering and the resources required to treat and rehabilitate the survivors. The striking prevalence of the disease demanded research, and the research showed that the higher a person's cholesterol the more likely it was that a stroke or heart attack would follow. This, in

THE TRUE CAUSES OF MOST HUMAN SUFFERING ARE YET TO BE DISCOVERED.

turn, led to the knowledge that a diet high in fat caused an elevation in cholesterol levels. This is not news today, but at the time it was a revelation.

The American Heart Association was formed in an effort to turn the tide of suffering. They proposed we follow the pyramid diet. This diet features fatty and oily foods (such as meats, eggs, nuts, and dairy products) as the least common source of calories, and the starchy foods (such as breads, grains, pasta, legumes, fruits, and starchy vegetables, such as potatoes) as the most common source of calories.

It has taken many years, but now the low-fat, pyramid-based diet has become deeply ingrained in the American way of life. "Don't eat that; it has a lot of fat," or "I'll have the low-fat yogurt; it's better for your heart," is heard daily. Everywhere you turn today there are products labeled as low fat and healthful. Even America's junk food is labeled as low fat. The low-fat pyramid diet has permeated the very fabric of our lives. Do you not agree? So, if America has embraced the low-fat, heart-healthy diet, why are so many Americans still dying of heart disease and stroke?

The answer is quite simple. When we strictly follow a refined, low-fat diet, we tend to stay hungry. And since we cannot have another serving of meat or fatty foods, we fill up on sweet desserts or starchy snacks. Or our hunger sends us to a fast-food restaurant, where we pack in a high-fat, highly-refined meal. We are not fulfilling our essential fatty acid, protein, and nutrient requirements with this approach, and our hunger is never satisfied. We exceed our caloric limit for the day, and the extra calories from desserts, sodas and starchy snacks are converted to cholesterol in our bloodstreams and fat on our frames.

Protein and the essential fatty acid oils are vital components of our diet. We cannot make these elements from sugar or starch. They must be present with each meal. If not present, our bodies will crave them and this craving cannot be satisfied by starch. If you try, you will gain weight and raise your cholesterol level. As your weight increases, so does your hunger. That's right, overweight people are hungrier than thin people! Adipose (fat) cells make hormones that drive hunger. And to complicate matters further, an overweight person burns fewer calories, pound per pound, than a thin person. Adipose cells have a slow metabolic rate compared to muscle and organ tissue.

As these metabolic stresses accumulate our bodies become unable to make sufficient quantities of critical metabolic intermediates, known as conditionally essential nutrients; deficiencies of which greatly aggravate cardiovascular disease. Coenzyme Q10, L-carnitine and D-ribose are all conditionally essential nutrients and their levels are frequently suboptimal in heart disease patients and our heart medications do nothing to increase their levels.

We have created a system that perpetuates obesity and heart disease by insisting we eat low-fat foods that are high in starch, foods that are too often refined and incapable of meeting our nutritional needs. And our high-tech methods of treating heart disease do nothing to restore nutrients and key metabolic intermediates to their optimal health promoting levels.

As explained, by following a high-starch diet, many tend to overeat, resulting in a metabolic conversion of starch to cholesterol and fat. It is this tendency to overeat carbohydrates that has caused the pyramid diet to fail for so many. It is also one of the reasons why so many diabetics with poor blood-sugar control have a high cholesterol level and are at such high risk for heart disease. High blood-sugar levels raise cholesterol.

It is a common misconception that dietary cholesterol, or the cholesterol in the foods we eat, dramatically raises blood cholesterol. It does not. Most of the cholesterol in your diet is digested as a food. The liver makes cholesterol from sugars, starches, fats, and oils, and it is very important for the body's many functions. Cholesterol is the basic building block for most hormones such as estrogen, progesterone, testosterone, and cortisol. It is an integral part of what we are. If we do not ingest enough cholesterol, our livers will manufacture it from oils, fats, starches, and sugars.

The types of oils, fats, starches, and sugars consumed greatly influence how much cholesterol the body makes and its overall health. Refined white sugar, grains, and corn syrup raise the blood's glucose quickly, providing an abundant source of energy for the production of fat and cholesterol. Whole grains provide the required vitamins and minerals to process their contained energy, and they release their energy slowly, thereby resisting their conversion to fat and cholesterol by the body's enzyme systems. The "good oils" in our diet, called polyunsaturated fatty acids, lower LDL-cholesterol (the "bad" cholesterol). Triglycerides, raise HDL-cholesterol (the "good" cholesterol), maintain cell wall integrity, inhibit platelet aggregation and abnormal blood clotting, stabilize blood sugar, and lower the incidence of some types of cancer, along with playing a role in a multitude of biochemical reactions. We cannot live without these fatty-acid oils; we need a daily source of them in our diet.

There is much confusion surrounding the source and use of polyunsaturated fatty acid oils in diet. Doctors and scientists make this concept sound very complicated, but it is not. The essential fatty acids are of two types, omega-3 fatty acids, including alpha-linolenic acid and eicosapentaenoic acid (EPA) and omega-6 fatty acids, including gamma-linolenic and linoleic acids. Among the most beneficial omega-3 fatty acids is EPA. Cold ocean fish oil is the single most abundant source of EPA. However, there are many vegetable sources of alpha-linolenic acid (an omega-3 fatty acid) that the body's enzyme systems convert to EPA, including flaxseed, canola, walnut, hemp, black currant seed, and perilla oils. Omega-6 fatty acids can be found in raw nuts and seeds, including borage, grape, sesame, black currant and hemp seed, legumes (beans), evening primrose, and soy bean oil. Conjugated linoleic acid (CLA) is an excellent source of omega-6 fatty acids. CLA is found in ruminant's (cow, goat, bison, deer, and elk) meat and milk fat, including butter, cream, cottage cheese, buttermilk, and yogurt.

The beneficial oils and fats of plants, fish, and ruminant source CLA are liquid oils at room temperature. The complex biochemistry of beneficial fatty acids can be condensed into this simple statement: if the fat or oil is liquid and from fish, plants, seeds, nuts or ruminants, make it a part of your diet and supplements. This liquid state is a chemical property of the beneficial polyunsaturated fatty acids and an easy-to-identify characteristic for laymen and scientists alike.

Harmful fats and saturated oils (hydrogenated vegetable oils) tend to be solid at room temperature or are added to highly processed, prepackaged foods, and thus easy to identify and avoid. Solid animal fats and hydrogenated oils, of any source, are fats to avoid.

A diversity of ocean fish, seeds, nuts, and their oils, along with vegetable oils and lean beef, mutton, goat, deer, and elk, along with their butter, cream, buttermilk, and cottage cheese will supply benefits associated with the omega-3 and omega-6 fatty acids. They all have beneficial properties. Pour vegetable oils onto salads. Take them as supplements. Consume lean ruminant meats and their fermented milk and milk-fat products. Their use is a consistent feature of the healthy and vital. These essential fatty acid oils actually lessen the risk of heart disease. Fats, such as solid beef and pork fat, and hydrogenated oils, such as margarine, are solid at room temperature and are easily converted to cholesterol and other damaging substances. Excessive amounts are a consistent feature of the unhealthy person's diet.

It is wise to limit red meat fat. Make red meats as lean as possible, but do not be afraid of them. Meat contains high levels of essential nutrients. Include fowl as a source of protein; however, fowl fat is no better for you than beef or pork fat. The single best source of protein and essential fatty acids is fish, particularly cold ocean fish, such as salmon, cod, and tuna. Try to eat more fish, but if this is not your cup of tea, take fish oils as a supplement on a daily basis. Your heart will thank you.

Limit starch intake. Protein, fats, and oils can be converted to glucose, or blood sugar. Starchy and sugary foods are the least nutritious of all foods, especially in the common forms of refined white flour, white sugar, white rice, and potatoes. These are the food sources to limit.

The pyramid diet is difficult to follow, and for it to be effective, the foods cannot be refined. Eating nature's whole foods is the answer. Nature provides more than enough vitamins, minerals, and fatty acids in complete whole grains to meet our needs. Do not believe for a minute that the vitamin solution put into the box of refined cereal, pasta, or white bread makes up for the refinement of the flour.

Eat raw nuts and seeds as snacks and tart fruits and berries for dessert. This is what the body is actually craving. Build meals around essential protein and fatty acid requirements. Include frequent servings of the variously colored, garden-fresh raw vegetables. The starches will take care of themselves.

Now that I have made you nice and comfortable, I'm going to make you uneasy again. Have you ever noticed that when you are confused about a problem, you often do not have enough information to make a good decision? Could there be another piece to the puzzle of heart disease? Yes, there is. In recent years, researchers have found silent inflammation throughout the entire body is a major cause of cardiovascular disease. This inflammation is often caused by chronic low-grade infections or imbalances of the micro-flora (bacteria) of the airways, urinary tract or the gastrointestinal tract. Perhaps this is why half of the people who have heart attacks have normal cholesterol levels. If so, would an antibiotic be the answer? If an antibiotic were the answer, the heart attack issues would have been solved years ago. Americans already take too many antibiotics. The answer, in part is in restoring the delicate balance of microbes that reside on and within each and every one of us.

MOST AMERICANS DON'T REALIZE HOW STRONG AN INFLUENCE THE PHARMACEUTICAL INDUSTRY HAS ON THE METHODS OF AMERICAN DOCTORS.

There are many other risk factors for heart disease and stroke. Cholesterol is but one. American allopathic medicine has focused its heart-disease prevention efforts on lowering cholesterol because the blood cholesterol level can be manipulated by antidote medication. To do only this is shortsighted and incomplete. To understand and formulate an effective program of prevention or treatment of heart disease consider the list of known risk factors.

MAJOR RISK FACTORS FOR HEART DISEASE AND STROKE

1. Smoking

2. Diabetes

3. Hypertension

4. Sedentary lifestyle

5. Elevated cholesterol level

6. Total body inflammation

MINOR RISK FACTORS FOR HEART DISEASE AND STROKE

7. Male gender

8. Female gender after menopause

9. Family history of heart disease and stroke

10. Obesity and fat distribution pattern. Abdominal fat distribution is a greater risk than hip fat distribution.

11. High-stress job

12. Aggressive personality

13. Malnutrition

14. Poor dental health

15. Excessive alcohol intake (greater than two drinks daily)

16. Any coexisting disease that creates a chronic stress

17. Intestinal infection with Helicobacter pylori

18. Lung or reproductive organ infection with Chlamydia

19. History of drug abuse

20. Chemical exposure

21. Elevated blood homocysteine level

22. Any medication that adversely affects blood cholesterol and lipid levels, such as diuretics and beta-blockers (some of the most commonly used medications for the treatment of hypertension and heart disease)

23. Low blood potassium and magnesium levels

24. Refined diet low in fiber

25. Depression

26. Low antioxidant blood level

27. Low essential fatty acid blood level

28. Elevated fibrinogen blood level

29. Low high-density lipoprotein blood level

30. High low-density lipoprotein blood level

31. High triglyceride blood level

32. Elevated C-reactive protein blood level

33. Probably many more factors yet to be understood

From the above list, it is obvious why every other heart attack victim has cholesterol within normal levels. Heart disease is a complicated disease process affected by many factors, 75 percent of which can be influenced for the better with healthy lifestyle practices. The Ten-State Nutritional Survey study showed that at least half of all Americans are consuming a diet deficient in the nutrients needed to counter known heart attack risk factors.

The arteries are under constant attack from various offenders. This is a normal part of life that continues without your being aware of it. If proper nutrition and lifestyle practices are in place, the body heals these insults without event. The deposit of cholesterol into arteries is the result of the body's attempt to cover and heal the injured artery. This is a normal "band-aid" attempt to seal off the injury. If the system has what it needs to repair the initial insult, the "wound" is much less likely to progress to a blockage of blood flow through the artery. Does it make sense to only remove the "band-aid" by artificially lowering the cholesterol? Much more is required. The purpose of holistic treatment is to provide these essential elements.

Let us consider my Aunt Lucille. At the time of her death Aunt Lucille was ninety-four years of age. She was a near-vegetarian all of her life. She consumed meat infrequently, and when she did, it was lean, and it was never pork. She never passed up a chance to eat ocean fish. She walked almost daily. She consumed soy products and eggs on a daily basis. She never smoked or drank and had no significant health problems, other than what you would expect for a woman of her seniority, until her death. She had a strong faith and took life as it came. Throughout her life she never had a stroke or a heart attack, and she had a total cholesterol level of over 450 for her entire life.

Do not think Aunt Lucille is an isolated case. There are tens of thousands of healthy, vibrant people with similar histories.

WHEN GIVEN WHAT IT NEEDS, THE HUMAN BODY IS CAPABLE OF GREAT THINGS.

If you have multiple risk factors for heart disease and stroke, or have already had a heart attack or stroke, work closely with your doctor and consider adding the following recommendations to your daily blood vessel-wise preventive plan.

1. Sheldon Saul Hendler, Ph.D., M.D. *Physicians' Desk Reference for Nutritional Supplements.* 1st Edition.

2. Michael Murray, N.D. and Joseph Pizzorno, N.D.; *Encyclopedia of Natural Medicine.* Revised 2nd Edition.

3. Phyllis A. Balch, CNC and James F. Balch, M.D., *Prescription for Nutritional Healing.* 3rd Edition.

Rx _____

RECOMMENDATIONS FOR CARDIOVASCULAR HEALTH

1. If you have a greatly elevated cholesterol level or have gained weight, the HEALING DIET will provide better results than the American Heart Association Pyramid

low-fat diet. If you choose to follow the American Heart Association Pyramid low-fat diet you must consume only whole foods, unprocessed, and unrefined. You cannot eat a low-fat diet five days of the week and then indulge in high-fat and refined carbohydrate foods on the weekends. I do not recommend the American Heart Association Diet due to the difficulty in following it and the poor results it provides.

2. After you have lost the added weight or reduced your cholesterol level, advance to the TRANSITIONAL DIET and then onto the DIET FOR THE REST OF YOUR LIFE as tolerated. You may stay with any level of the diets at your choosing if it is controlling your cholesterol and you feel well.

3. Juice with carrots and low-starch vegetables for lycopene and lutein.

4. Include frequent servings of legumes and soy products as they have been shown to decrease heart attack risk.

5. Remember that fats that are solid at room temperature should be avoided, whether they originate from animal or hydrogenated vegetable sources. They must be limited with either plan. The fatty acid oils that are liquid at room temperature are essential to both

plans and should be consumed daily. Pour them onto your salads and low-starch vegetables.

6. If you have evidence of a fungal infection of any type (fungal toenails, dandruff, athlete's foot, or recurrent yeast infections, etc.), you will achieve best results by correcting the condition with the HEALING DIET and the measures outlined in the chapter on fungal diseases.

7. Soy isoflavones: 200 mg daily: may be used by men and women.

8. Fish or flaxseed oil with borage seed oil: 2-4 grams a day of each and consume cold water ocean fish twice a week.

9. Vitamin E: 400–800 I.U. daily.

10. Vitamin C: 1 gram daily.

11. Multiple mineral that contains calcium 1–2 grams, magnesium 500–1,000 mg, selenium 200 micrograms, zinc. 25 mg, and a source of the trace minerals, such as sea kelp, 1–2 grams daily.

12. B-Complex: 50 mg up to 3 times daily.

13. Vitamin A: with mixed carotenoids 10,000 I.U. daily.

14. Protein supplement from naturally occurring whole protein source 2–4 grams daily to assure essential amino acid requirements.

15. High potency multiple vitamin, mineral and amino acid powder: 1 tbs daily in water may be used in place of numbers 10–15.

16. Coenzyme Q10/L-carnitine: 30 mg/250 mg 2-4 gel caps daily. Many heart patients take up to 1000 mg of coenzyme Q10 and 1500 mg of L-carnitine daily without difficulty. If you take a cholesterol-lowering drug the importance of supplementing Coenzyme Q10 doubles.

17. D-ribose: 5-10 grams twice daily. D-ribose is a naturally occurring carbohydrate used by our bodies to produce ATP; the source of energy for the heart.

18. Garlic: 3–4 grams daily. Also include garlic in your daily diet.

19. Grape seed-extracted oligomeric proanthocyanidins (OPC) with at least 95% active component purity: 100–300 mg daily.

20. Grape skin-extracted resveratrol: 50 mg daily.

21. Beta glucan: 3 mg 1–2 capsules daily. If you have had a heart attack or stroke, or if you have multiple risk factors, take beta glucan: 10 mg 1–2 capsules daily.

22. IP6: 100 mg daily.

23. Noni juice: 1–4 oz daily.

24. Glucomannan fiber: 575 mg 4-6 capsules daily with a large glass of water. Psyllium: 1 tbs in water daily is another fiber option.

25. Probiotics with fructo-oligosaccharides: 1 tablet daily.

26. Gingko biloba: 240 mg daily. Do not take gingko if you are taking a "blood thinner" such as Coumadin (warfarin).

27. Astragalus: 500 mg up to 3 capsules 3 times daily.

28. Exercise for at least 20 minutes 4–5 times a week. A simple rule of thumb to consider if you have a

heart condition: you are pushing too hard if you cannot carry on a conversation while exercising without gasping for breath. Clearance from your doctor prior to exercise is always a good idea.

29. Reduce coffee and soda intake, and consider drinking tea.

30. Reduce salt intake. Do not add salt, and be aware of foods' salt content. Nature provides you adequate sodium in whole foods. Prepackaged foods almost always have too much sodium.

31. Remember that controlling blood pressure, blood sugar, and weight is as important in preventing heart attacks as controlling cholesterol level.

32. If your heart condition is complicated by diabetes refer to Chapter 14 and incorporate the recommendations for diabetes in your plan for wellness.

Richard L. Becker, .D.O.

IF THE DOCTOR SAYS, "THIS WON'T HURT A BIT,"

HE IS REFERRING TO HIS PAIN LEVEL,

AND YOU HAD BETTER BRACE YOURSELF.

17

ALLERGIES, ECZEMA, AND ASTHMA

We all know someone who suffers from allergies, eczema, or asthma. These common afflictions can make life miserable, and asthma can be life-threatening. The varied conditions go by many names—allergic rhinitis, chronic sinusitis, hay fever, spring fever, seasonal or perennial rhinitis, dermatitis, eczema, asthma, and obstructive pulmonary disease, to name a few. But all these conditions have in common an underlying, abnormal, immune reaction to various stimuli in the environment or diet.

DOCTORS AND MEDICATIONS SAVE LIVES ON A DAILY BASIS . . . SIGNIFICANTLY MORE PEOPLE'S LIVES ARE SAVED THAN HARMED.

These conditions may occur for only a few days of the year or they may be daily afflictions. Symptoms include sinus drainage, sneezing, itchy and watery eyes, coughing, wheezing, ear popping and pain, red itchy and flaky skin with an unusual propensity toward depression and fatigue. These conditions can simply wear you out! Some allergy sufferers' conditions are complicated by asthma and eczema. Still others find their intestinal tracts involved. Burning stomach pain, diarrhea and altered bowel flora are not unusual for severe allergy sufferers.

When sinuses and the respiratory tract are under constant assault, tissues swell and mucus accumulates, followed by sinus pressure and pain. Many allergy sufferers develop chronic sinus or lung infections, which are difficult to cure. Fungal infections of the sinuses frequently complicate allergic disorders and the well-intended but ineffective treatment of these infections with antibiotics further disturbs the delicate balance of microbes in the intestinal tract.

An asthmatic's wheeze may not be due to allergies. An infection from any source—viral, bacterial, or fungal—may also induce wheezing. Pollution and high ozone levels can also play a part in the malady. The induction of airway spasm, or wheezing, may be for various reasons, but the same physiologic response occurs in all and can be affected positively by the same corrective measures.

When a person suffers from allergies, doctors call the process immediate hypersensitivity of the IgE variety. This simply means that your body is creating antibodies to protein particles that ordinarily would not harm you. For example, antibodies combine with ragweed pollen proteins and initiate an immune reaction that makes you miserable. It must be understood that this propensity is genetically programmed and is present to some degree in all of us. Allergic reactions are most active in the developing years of childhood and adolescence and they normally calm by adulthood.

Yet some people continue to react well into their adult and senior years. Some unfortunate souls have inherited a strong tendency to react to harmless proteins in the air, but they are a minority. Most do not have genetic propensity, but they still continue to cough, sneeze, hack, and wheeze. Time and again, the doctor prescribes blocking antihistamines, immune-suppressive steroid sprays, creams and injections, antibiotics, and adrenaline-like substances to open airways.

When this process continues over time, it creates a major stress in the patient's life. The condition becomes a beast, which requires stronger and stronger medications to control. What can we do to help the chronic allergy, sinus, eczema, and asthma sufferer?

The answer to this dilemma lies not in the suppression of allergy symptoms, but in correcting the underlying disorder. The disorder I speak of is usually in the intestines and is based in nutritional deficiencies, altered intestinal micro- flora and unwanted side effects of medications. If essential minerals, vitamins and conditionally essential nutrients are even marginally low the genetic propensity to react to allergens and pollutants is amplified. If allergies and asthma are left untreated, immune reactions further deplete precious vitamins and minerals. Unfortunately, the medications frequently used for allergies and asthma can ultimately create an imbalance in the intestinal tract that further perpetuates the syndrome. This imbalance must be corrected if we are to succeed in the treatment of allergies, asthma and chronic sinusitis.

THE MORE MEDICATION YOU TAKE THE MORE MEDICATION YOU WILL NEED.

If you have had enough coughing, hacking, sneezing, and wheezing, then follow these corrective measures, and, with time, I know you will be amazed!

ALLERGY, ECZEMA, AND ASTHMA CORRECTION PROTOCOL

Not every sinusitis, allergy, eczema, or asthma sufferer will need everything on this list. For many, the vitamin and mineral, as well as dietary, recommendations will be enough. Some, however, will need the complete program. The abrupt onset of allergies in adulthood can be a sign of a serious underlying health condition. Fortunately, this is not a common occurrence. If you have faithfully followed this program for 30 to 60 days without improvement, see your doctor for a complete physical.

Rx _____

RECOMMENDATIONS FOR ALLERGIES, ECZEMA, AND ASTHMA

1. Absolute restriction of refined sugars, grains, and altered fats (hydrogenated oils such as margarine).

2. If you have any evidence of a fungal disorder such as chronic sinusitis, recurrent yeast infections, dandruff, fungal toenails, jock itch, athlete's foot, or have taken multiple rounds of antibiotics or steroids, including birth control pills, you must incorporate into your plan the HEALING DIET and the measures listed to treat Candida, yeast, and fungal infections. The simple addition of oil

of oregano and olive leaf extract to your plan may make all the difference in your health and vitality.

3. No carbonated beverages of any type. Reduce coffee and tea intake and drink 1/2 ounce of chlorine-free water per pound of body weight daily.

4. Increase low-starch vegetables and tart fruits.

5. Vary your diet. Do not eat the same thing day after day. Consider instituting an elimination diet to determine which foods you may be reacting too.

6. Avoid exposure to offending allergens if possible. If your house has a mold problem, the mold must be eradicated. Use a dust mask while mowing the yard, if you react to grass.

7. Vitamin C: 1–2 grams daily.

8. Vitamin B-5: Pantothenic Acid, 300 mg daily.

9. Vitamin B-6: Pyridoxine, 100 mg daily.

10. Vitamin B-12: Cyanocobalamine, 1000 micrograms sublingual daily.

11. Vitamin E: 400 I.U. daily.

12. Calcium: 1 gram daily.

13. Magnesium: 500 mg daily.

14. Zinc: 25 mg daily.

15. High potency multiple vitamin, mineral and amino acid powder: 1 tbs daily in water may be used in place of numbers 7–14.

16. Fish or flaxseed oil with borage seed oil: 1–2 grams of each daily.

17. Noni juice: 2–3 oz daily on an empty stomach.

18. Beta glucan: 10 mg, 1 capsule twice daily with Noni juice on an empty stomach.

19. Quercetin: 500 mg daily.

20. Coenzyme Q10/L-carnitine: 30 mg/250 mg 1-2 gel caps daily.

21. Oligomeric proanthocyanidins (OPC) with at least 95% active component purity: 100 mg daily.

22. Bee pollen-propolis-royal jelly: harvested near your home in powder, granule, or opened capsule form. Start with 2–4 granules or a small amount of powder under the tongue, double the dose every 6 hours until 1 tsp of granules or powder, then 1 tsp or capsule daily thereafter. (CAUTION: One person out of 240 is extremely allergic to bee pollen. By starting with a low dose and increasing slowly you will minimize the risk of reaction. Do not use any bee product if you know you are allergic to bee stings.)

23. Probiotics with fructo-oligosaccharides: 1-2 tablets daily for 90 days then 1-2 tablets weekly thereafter.

24. Glucomannan fiber: 575 mg 4-6 capsules daily with a large glass of water. Psyllium: 1 tbs in water daily is another fiber option.

24. Echinacea (freeze-dried root): 325–650 mg twice daily if recurrent infections complicate your condition.

25. Sinus-wash with grapefruit seed extract and oregano: 1-2 drops or puffs per nostril 1-2 times daily. This simple remedy is immensely helpful for chronic sinusitis.

26. Homeopathic combination allergy drops or tablets: the products contents should correlate with your

seasonal reactivity. For example: spring reactions—trees; summer reactions—grasses; late summer to fall reactions— ragweed and weeds; all year reactions— house dust, mold, and dander. Follow instructions on the bottle.

27. If you have asthma, always keep an asthma inhaler close by for emergencies. Over time the need for this rescue medication will diminish.

28. Skin emollient containing Noni and beta glucan: apply to eczema-affected areas as often as needed. This soothing cream calms irritated skin without any steroids.

29. Allergy testing and shots that desensitize the patient can be extremely helpful. They may, however, require up to 2 to 3 years of weekly injections in some extreme cases before the patient perceives an improvement. (Most, however, benefit within 6 to 8 months.)

Richard L. Becker, .D.O.

IF A PHARMACIST'S JOB WERE ONLY COUNTING

PILLS AND TYPING PILL BOTTLE LABELS HE WOULD

GET HIS DIPLOMA AFTER FIRST GRADE.

18

BENIGN PROSTATE ENLARGEMENT

No words can describe the trouble an enlarged prostate can cause a man. Up from sleep three or four times a night with an urgent need to empty the bladder only to dribble, being constantly aware of the closest restroom, or pain and burning on elimination are all but a small sampling of the troubles that are possible.

PAIN AND SUFFERING ARE NOT A NORMAL PART OF AGING.

Unfortunately, this is a far too common affliction in men over fifty years of age. The medical community considers enlargement of the prostate normal, believing that the gland doubles in size every decade after fifty years of age. Just as pain is not a normal part of aging, dramatic enlargement of the prostate is not normal and can be helped with some simple holistic measures.

There are four basic afflictions of the prostate gland: infection, inflammation, benign enlargement, and cancer. All four can be present at once, alone, or in any combination of the four.

The prostate gland sits at the base of the bladder. Through its structure flows the urethra or the tube that empties the bladder. If the gland becomes abnormally large, free flow of urine becomes compromised.

Under a microscope, the prostate resembles a sponge. It is an organ affected by testosterone, estrogen, and progesterone, just as a woman's uterus is. Men who are balding frequently have an extra enzyme that converts testosterone to another more powerful testosterone—dihydrotestosterone. This phenomenon misaligns the testosterone-to-progesterone balance, leading to enlargement of the prostate to troublesome size. If these unfortunate men also have a propensity for high cholesterol and triglycerides they are at a greater risk because this combination causes dramatic enlargement and congestion of this sponge-like gland. However, you do not need to be balding or have a high cholesterol level to be troubled by your prostate. The delicate hormone balance needed for proper prostate health can be altered by an abnormal colonization of the intestinal tract by yeast and bacteria. These organisms have the ability to make hormones and hormone-like substances that can enlarge the prostate gland.

MEN, IF YOU THINK YOU HAVE IT ROUGH AT THE DOCTOR'S OFFICE, HAVE A TALK WITH YOUR WIFE ABOUT THE CHALLENGES OF CHILDBIRTH.

Since the prostate gland is difficult to reach, you will need the help of your doctor to accurately diagnose the problem. Once this has been achieved, and enlargement of the prostate has been confirmed, keep these simple measures in mind as this protocol has helped many men to restore normal urinary flow.

Rx

RECOMMENDATIONS FOR BENIGN PROSTATE ENLARGEMENT

1. If you have taken multiple rounds of antibiotics or have been on antibiotics for a prolonged period of time, for any reason, have an elevated cholesterol and triglyceride level, have had prostate infections or been on steroid or hormone therapy, for best results follow the HEALING DIET until better. Then advance through the TRANSITIONAL DIET to the DIET FOR THE REST OF YOUR LIFE as

tolerated. Include pumpkin seeds, fresh garden salads with a variety of colored vegetables and 6-8 oz of pomegranate juice in your daily diet for overall prostate health. Also include the spices turmeric, ginger, rosemary, oregano leaf and royal jelly in your diet or as a supplement as they calm inflammation.

2. Probiotics with fructo-oligosaccharides: 1-2 tablets daily for 6 months then 1-2 tablets weekly thereafter.

3. Olive leaf extract: 100 mg twice daily.

4. Pau d'arco: 500 mg 2 capsules twice daily.

5. Oil of Oregano: 5–10 drops in water or 1-2 gel caps twice daily.

6. Saw Palmetto berry extract oil: 160 mg twice daily. The longer you stay on saw palmetto the better your response to the herb will be.

7. Pygeum bark extract: 50 mg twice daily.

8. Wild yam root extract: 275–550 mg daily.

9. If after 45 days insufficient progress has been made,

add progesterone cream 1/2 tsp to the inner thigh or forearm daily.

10. Flaxseed oil: 3–8 grams daily. Flaxseed oil is the preferred omega-3 fatty acid source over fish oil for prostate disorders due to flaxseed's high lignan content.

11. Zinc: 50 mg daily.

12. B-Complex: 50 mg twice daily.

13. Calcium: 1 gram daily.

14. Magnesium: 500 mg daily.

15. Selenium: 100 micrograms daily.

16. Sea kelp: 1 gram daily.

17. High potency multiple vitamin, mineral and amino acid powder: 1 tbs daily may be substituted for numbers 11–16.

18. Noni juice: 1-2 oz twice daily.

19. Beta glucan: 10 mg 1 or 2 capsules daily if your condition is complicated by prostate infections.

20. Drink 1/2 oz chlorine-free water, per pound of body weight daily.

Richard L. Becker, .D.O.

A BOY IS DETERMINED TO AVOID WORK;

A MAN WORKS WITH DETERMINATION.

19

MENOPAUSE MANAGEMENT
THE NATURAL WAY

Ladies, have you ever wondered what the world of medicine would be like if women had historically dominated the medical profession? There is no doubt that things would be much different. Certainly one of the things that would be different is how doctors manage menopause and its varied incapacitating complaints.

I can think of no other subject that draws such heated debate. Every week there is a press

MOST OF THE GROUNDBREAKING STUDIES AND NEW DISCOVERIES REPORTED IN THE NEWSPAPER ARE AT LEAST TWENTY YEARS OLD . . . . HOW ELSE DO YOU FILL A NEWSPAPER ON A SLOW NEWS DAY?

release that conflicts with the last press release on the effects of estrogen and progesterone. Does estrogen cause cancer? Does it really prevent osteoporosis? Will I have a heart attack if I take estrogen? Will I gain weight and raise my blood pressure? What type of hormone is the best? Should I take the horse estrogen my doctor recommends? Or, perhaps, take the new synthetic estrogen just patented by a large pharmaceutical company? If I still have a uterus will I need to take estrogen and progesterone? Will my periods return? WHAT A MESS!

To help you recapture control of your life, let us use some common sense to understand the process of menopause and formulate a safe and effective plan.

Most women are born with a large number of viable eggs. Starting during puberty, the normal process of hormone peaks and valleys causes one egg to be released mid-cycle for fertilization. Eventually the viable eggs are depleted. This is the time of menopause, which arrives for most women at age fifty but can start as early as thirty or as late as sixty-five.

During the change, but before the eggs are completely depleted, there is a period of time in many women when ovulation becomes irregular and normal cycling of hormones becomes greatly amplified, creating strange hormonal swings. A woman may not have a period for several months, followed by a massive flow. This difficult time is called perimenopause and is characterized by hot flashes, mood swings, irritability, loss of sex drive, dry skin and mucous membranes, hastened signs of aging, headaches, night sweats, vaginal dryness and itching, and disturbed sleep.

Menopause can also be brought on early by surgically removing the uterus and ovaries—a procedure called hysterectomy. Even if the ovaries are not removed, menopause may still be initiated due to a compromised blood flow to the ovaries during a hysterectomy.

The disabling symptoms of menopause are brought about by the wide fluctuation of hormones that frequently occur during this challenging time. If hormone swings can be steadied and stabilized, symptoms of menopause can be greatly improved.

When a woman is in the throes of symptomatic menopause, she and her loved ones are highly motivated to find relief. The fastest and strongest relief available is either synthesized or true hormones, in large doses. The demand for quick relief has created a huge business opportunity for doctors and the pharmaceutical industry. Unfortunately, only synthetic hormones, which are foreign to humans, or human hormones, produced by unique methods of extracting, can be patented and thus profitable for pharmaceutical companies.

While providing quick relief, over time this approach leads to greatly elevated hormone levels, which, in turn, lead to serious complications, such as heart disease, hypertension, weight gain, and cancer. Herein lies the problem for the symptomatic, menopausal woman. The only help made available to her has often been these foreign or extracted hormones, which come with all-too-frequent debilitating side effects, sometimes occurring months to years after the hormones have been started. Fortunately, taking hormones is not the only option for menopausal women today.

We all know someone who has breezed through menopause without a symptom, never taking one dose of hormones. In Japan, menopausal symptoms are rare. In fact, the Japanese language has no word for hot flash, and this observation has led to scientific research that you should know about.

First, though hormone levels drop with menopause, ovaries, adrenal glands, specialized sweat glands, and fat cells all continue to make hormones. Secondly, if the production of hormones by these structures can be improved and normal low levels of menopausal hormones supported with non-hormone plant extracts and essential nutrients, the menopausal transition can be greatly eased. The key is keeping the body's system in charge. No skilled doctor or hormone of human manufacture can regulate your hormone levels as safely and effectively as your own healthy set of organs, even if you have had a hysterectomy.

The soy plant contains estrogen-like substances called isoflavones that partially activate hormone receptors without over-stimulating the target organ. The Japanese consume large amounts of soy, thereby alleviating menopausal symptoms. Soy isoflavones have NO TRUE ESTROGEN HORMONE WHATSOEVER and are incapable of over-stimulating the estrogen receptors. Over-stimulation is the reason synthetic and extracted true hormones come with such a list of side effects. Over-stimulation is to be avoided at all cost.

Wild yam contains a substance called disogenin, which does for progesterone what soy does for estrogen, partially activating the progesterone receptors while normalizing adrenal gland function with NO TRUE PROGESTERONE HORMONE WHATSOEVER. Likewise, this substance is incapable of over-stimulating the receptors. When taken together, wild yam and soy extracts supply essential nutrients, which provide bone protection, cardiovascular protection, cancer protection, immune enhancement, mood support, hormone level stabilization, and a state of well-being, with no return of your periods. To achieve this end with true hormones, synthetic or otherwise, is extremely difficult. The body's hormone regulation system is complicated and difficult to manipulate with true hormones. Soy and yam extracts have a wide dosage range due to their non-hormone nature, providing remarkable safety.

Soy and yam extracts are so remarkable they can even be used for detoxification after an overdose of true hormones taken by prescription. Simply start the extracts and slowly over several weeks decrease the prescription hormone dose, being careful to avoid rapid withdrawal symptoms, which may make you return to taking hormone pills needlessly.

NATURE HOLDS THE ANSWER TO MOST OF OUR HEALTH NEEDS.

Not all male doctors are insensitive to the needs of women. It is really more about science than gender!

Put these simple holistic measures to work and in a few weeks you will be feeling better than ever.

Rx _____

RECOMMENDATIONS FOR MENOPAUSE MANAGEMENT

1. If you have been taking prescription hormone replacement therapy (HRT) and have been diagnosed with virtually any syndrome of failing health

including hypertension, weight gain, autoimmune disease, depression, or anxiety since starting hormone therapy, follow the HEALING DIET to lose weight and help normalize your system. Include in your diet the cruciferous vegetables and extracts (cabbage, broccoli, brussels sprouts, cauliflower, bok choy, and kale) as they contain indole-3 carbinol. The cruciferous plants and their extracts are helpful in countering the toxic effects of HRT.

2. If you have been taking prescription HRT and have decided to stop this therapy, start the recommendations listed below while still taking HRT and slowly decrease the dose of HRT over several weeks as tolerated. The human body adapts to external sources of hormones even if the dose is too high. Abruptly stopping HRT may cause withdrawal-like symptoms, impelling you to restart the hormones needlessly. Reducing HRT dosages slowly over 4 to 8 weeks by alternate-day dosing and dosage reduction, while following the recommendations listed below, will spare you unnecessary side effects.

3. Soy isoflavones: 125–250 mg daily. If you have been taking HRT start the soy isoflavones dosage at the higher dose while you decrease HRT to help ease the transition off hormones. Once the transition is

complete and you are doing well, use the least soy isoflavones to maintain your sense of well-being. If you have not been taking HRT and are experiencing unpleasant menopause symptoms, you may also use a higher dosage to ease your symptoms, then decrease as tolerated.

4. Wild yam extract: 275–550 mg with 10 percent diosgenin. As with soy isoflavones dosages, if you have been taking HRT, start the wild yam dosage at the higher dose while you decrease the HRT to help ease the transition off hormones. Once the transition is complete and you are doing well, use the least amount of wild yam to maintain your sense of well-being. If you have not been taking HRT and are experiencing debilitating menopause symptoms you may also use the higher dosage to ease your symptoms, then decrease as tolerated.

5. Indole-3 carbinol: 200-400 mg daily. As with soy isoflavones and wild yam, start the indole-3 carbinol at the higher dose while you decrease the HRT to help ease the transition off hormones or to quickly calm menopause symptoms. Once the transition is complete and you are doing well use the least amount to ease your symptoms.

6. Flaxseed oil: 1000 mg 2-4 gel caps daily. Flaxseed oil is the preferred omega-3 source over fish oil for menopausal symptoms due to its high lignan content.

7. Progesterone cream: 1/4 – 1/2 tsp applied to thin skin such as the inner arm or thigh as needed up to six times daily. During the transition off HRT, you may experience hot flashes and mood swings. Over the counter progesterone cream may be used to control these symptoms. By using progesterone cream instead of pills you will avoid the majority of liver side effects associated with oral hormone medication. Topical application of hormones lessens the dose necessary to achieve good results. Not every woman will need progesterone cream. But it can be a real lifesaver during the difficult transition time of discontinuing HRT and menopause.

8. Remember nature never provides only one hormone at a time; it uses sets of hormones so it is important for you to use soy, wild yam, indole-3 carbinol and flaxseed oil for the most effective control of your symptoms. None of these supplements are true hormones and all are very safe to use. To start, use only these plant extracts. If you have a bad reaction or fail to improve you can easily determine the ingredient to blame.

9. Calcium: up to 2 grams daily.

10. Magnesium: up to 1 gram daily.

11. Boron: 3 mg daily.

12. Copper: 3 mg daily.

13. Zinc: 25 mg daily.

14. Sea kelp: 1 gram daily for trace minerals.

15. B-complex: up to 3 times daily.

16. Vitamin A: 5,000 I.U. daily.

17. Vitamin C: 1 gram daily.

18. Beta-carotene: 10,000 I.U. daily.

19. Folic acid: 400 micrograms daily.

20. High potency multiple vitamin, mineral and amino acid powder: 1 tbs daily may be used in place of numbers 9-19.

21. Noni juice: 1-2 oz daily and 1 oz whenever a hot flash occurs as needed.

22. It is better to experience hot flashes for a time than take high doses of HRT. Unfortunately many of the more serious side effects of HRT may take years to develop. If after 60–90 days you are not on the road to wellness, see your doctor for saliva hormone level testing and consider HRT with BIO-IDENTICAL HORMONE REPLACEMENT THERAPY using only true human hormones.

23. The four-year period of menopause is the time of greatest bone loss for women. Refer to Chapter 23 on osteoporosis and incorporate the measures listed into your wellness plan. You will see the measures for osteoporosis and menopause are very similar.

Richard L. Becker, .D.O.

HUMAN DEVELOPMENT NEVER STOPS

FROM CRADLE TO GRAVE.

20

OBESITY

The citizens of the United States are overweight. Go to any public place and look around you. You will see countless people who are desperately fighting a losing battle with obesity. Hundreds of scientific studies have shown the dangers of being overweight, yet we continue to gain.

EVERY AMERICAN SHOULD BE TAKING AT LEAST A MULTIPLE VITAMIN AND MINERAL.

Some fifteen years ago I was reading an article in *National Geographic* magazine about the fiftieth anniversary of the attack on Pearl Harbor. They featured a picture of the San Diego Naval Recruiting Office on December 8, 1941. There was a long line of young men, stripped to their underwear, waiting for their military clearance physicals. These were healthy-appearing young men, lean and naturally muscular, the look created by hard physical labor, not by lifting weights in the gym. Not one of the nearly fifty men shown was in the slightest way overweight. Their eyes were clear and bright with the look of apprehension expected of those headed to war.

Next to the picture of the 1941 naval recruits was a picture of the same recruiting office in San Diego fifty years later with a similar line of young men. However, the naval recruits from 1991 were almost all overweight. The typical young man in this picture carried fifteen to twenty pounds of extra fat, and some carried far more. The occasional exception was at ideal weight. The contrast was striking and undeniable. The time span was only fifty years, yet the pictures spoke volumes of the changes modern times have brought and the problem is even worse now in the new millennia.

Since this article, I have observed the same phenomenon in countless historical photographs. I am sure you have also made this observation as have dozens of scientific studies that show the majority of Americans are now overweight or obese.

Since understanding a problem is the first step toward solving it, allow me to present a few historical and biological facts that will help you overcome your battle with obesity.

It is a common mistake made by doctors and patients to assume that an overweight person is well nourished. I recall a conversation with a physician of twenty-five-years experience who was fighting obesity and arthritis. I casually recommended he take B-Complex vitamins, as they are known to help both problems, to which he replied with a grin, "Just look at me, Richard; how could I be malnourished?"

Do not make the same mistake. The Hanes nutritional studies showed that up to 80 percent of America's population is consuming a diet low in at least one essential nutrient. This study included overweight people in its findings. It has been my experience that the vast majority of obese people are malnourished in some respect.

Malnourished people can gain weight by eating abnormal foods, foods that cannot meet their nutritional needs. Consider pica and pica-like syndromes mentioned earlier: the craving for abnormal foods. These cravings could be dirt, clay, chalk, ice, or an abnormally high number of starchy foods. These cravings always reflect a nutritional deficiency of some sort— of iron or some other essential nutrient. Yet the abnormal foods may bind any available iron in the intestines, thus preventing absorption of the deficient element and making the problem worse. Do not think this happens only to those deficient in iron, nor is it only displayed by eating dirt. It can happen in some form to anyone with any vitamin, mineral, protein, or essential fatty acid deficiency. The body's "inner doctor" becomes confused, giving us false signals of inappropriate hunger and cravings. When the system needs an essential element, all it can do is tell us with a sense of hunger and/or cravings. There is no computer screen in the brain that flashes before our eyes, "Eat iron-rich foods; you are deficient!" The cravings created by nutrient deficiencies are typically perceived as a need for starchy, sweet, or salty foods, which cannot fill the nutritional void, thus eating continues long past the point when caloric needs have been met.

Next consider the growing evidence that adipose tissue (fat cells) makes hormones, which drive the appetite and suppress metabolism. The primary function of the adipose cell is to retain energy during times of plenty so that there may be a ready source of fuel during the lean times. Fat cells do everything in their power to keep their reserve. This is but a fundamental adaptive response to the stresses of nature. Our surviving ancestors are those who withdrew from this bank of energy in miserly fashion during times of disease, famine, war, and migration. Just as a family may share appearance features, so may we share a propensity to be overweight.

This same ancestral human, to follow the example, never passed up an opportunity to eat. Frequent feedings were required to provide the energy spent on short bursts of hunting, gathering, and farming. Nor did he count calories or weigh the food he was about to eat. He ate his fill of berries as they ripened on the vine, knowing it would be a full year before they would be available again. He had no refrigeration or preservatives to keep his food fresh. When he killed a deer for meat, he consumed it as quickly as possible to maximize his intake before the meat spoiled. He covered wide ranges of land to find his food, thus continually exposing himself to a wide variety of the earth's foods and mineral elements. He also drank water not soda to quench his thirst.

Our ancestors' foods were never refined. All of his foods were whole with no part removed and his drink was chlorine-free water. Nature provides more than enough vitamins and minerals in complete organic foods to meet our needs.

In short, we are the surviving descendants of countless generations of humans who have physically worked hard on a daily basis just to eat, descendants of people who ate at every opportunity, never denying their hunger. We are people whose ancestors always ate complete, unrefined foods high in nutrient content. Any extra food, during times of plenty, was consumed and held as fat because it could not be preserved outside of the body as insurance for lean times.

But today things are different, are they not? Americans typically earn enough money in the first hour of work to pay for their entire day's food. They walk no farther than to the car and back. They satisfy their thirst with sugared sodas and sweet fruity drinks. They consume refined and preserved foods from artificially fertilized crops from around the world in any season.

I HAVE NEVER MET A SUCCESSFUL PERSON WHO WORKED ONLY A FORTY-HOUR WEEK.

They are continually told that a low-fat or new-age fad diet is the only beneficial way to eat. Their heritage dictates eating high oily and fatty meals at every opportunity and holding these calories as body fat for the lean times ahead. In today's world the lean times never come.

It is essential for any overweight person to acknowledge these fundamental ancestral driving forces and incorporate them into their modern lifestyles, if they would like to permanently change their pattern of obesity. Understand that glandular problems are rarely at the root of the problem, yet they occur as a consequence of it and can be effectively reversed with proper lifestyle measures. The time for discipline in weight loss is not in denying hunger but in making the right choices.

Before you say, "But, Dr.Becker, you are thin. How could you know how hard this is?" I, too, have struggled with my weight.

The recommendations listed below are a result of many years of helping myself and many patients regain exuberant vitality. Even while I write this passage, my teenage daughter, Tana, reminds me of how overweight I really am.

DESPITE MODERN SCIENTIFIC ADVANCEMENTS, THE FUNDAMENTAL NEEDS OF HUMANS HAVE REMAINED THE SAME FOR THOUSANDS OF YEARS.

Rx

RECOMMENDATIONS FOR WEIGHT LOSS AND WEIGHT GAIN PREVENTION

1. Always eat breakfast within thirty minutes of rising in the morning and never skip this meal. The meal may be light, but do not establish a pattern of skipping any meal. The remaining measures will become ineffective if this measure is ignored. Try to eat more calories early and fewer calories late in the day. Eat three meals a day and a snack. The snack should be protein-rich and low in natural sugar, such as mixed fresh nuts and a Granny Smith apple or berries. Skipping breakfast is the most common mistake made by those who are battling their weight.

2. You may replace 1 or 2 meals daily or a daily snack with a protein rich, low sugar meal replacement product (13 grams of sugars or less per serving). It is important however to continue to eat normal foods during your weight loss plan in order to maintain proper intestinal and organ function. For example:

   BREAKFAST: Meal replacement product.

   LUNCH: Well balanced meal using foods from the HEALING DIET.

   SNACK: Meal replacement product

   DINNER: Well balanced meal using foods from the HEALING DIET.

3. Immediately after a meal do not sit and rest. Get on your feet and move about or take a short walk. Exercise speeds up metabolism and prevents returning to the kitchen and snacking after the meal is complete.

4. Ignore ideal weight charts. These charts do not account for your unique body type. Your "inner doctor" will tell you when your weight is right.

5. Be prepared for a week of significant weight loss followed by a week or two of no loss in spite of every effort. This is a normal plateau of weight loss. The ideal pace for weight loss is no more than a pound a week. If it takes you a year to lose fifty pounds and you never suffer prolonged periods of hunger, eating whenever the need arises, how bad can that be? In fact, studies show this slow pattern of weight loss is the most likely to result in permanent loss.

6. Understand that many of the people in public places are not eating a normal diet, and for you to lose weight you must not eat like them, even if they are thin.

7. Surround yourself with healthy, active people. Understand that your image of enjoyable foods has been altered by the fast food industry, junk food snacks, and television advertisements, which create a notion that it is normal and even sexy to eat bad foods.

8. Eat only whole foods, as close to their natural state as possible.

9. If you are hungry eat, and eat all you want. But you must eat the right foods. Use discipline to choose the correct foods, not for denying hunger. For

example if you buy junk food and take it home, you will eat it.

10. Always do your grocery shopping on a full stomach. The junk and prepackaged food industry have taken considerable effort in designing food packaging and store placement to create an impulse to buy their products.

11. Shop from the outer aisle of the food store, avoiding the prepackaged and junk foods completely.

12. Try not to eat while watching television, reading, or working. Eating this way becomes entertainment, not a source of nourishment.

13. Slow down your pace of eating. Chew each bite slowly and deliberately, allowing ample time for a modest meal to raise your blood glucose and thus satisfy your hunger. The simple act of using a smaller food plate or bowl along with a smaller eating utensil to eat with will help you decrease your portion sizes and slow down your pace of eating.

14. When you eat out, choose a restaurant with healthful options. A cafeteria is a better choice because you can see the food options before ordering.

15. Observe people and their eating habits. Learn from their mistakes and their correct choices. Senior citizens have learned a lot in life, and in general their example is a healthful one.

16. Avoid artificial stimulants and drug appetite suppressants, as these measures do nothing to correct the underlying disorder of obesity. They certainly have their place in the management of obesity as a tool to help you get started, but they have NEVER been shown to permanently correct obesity.

17. Make every effort through dietary means to lose weight before you consult a surgeon for stomach bypass or Lap-Band surgery.

18. If you are on any type of hormone therapy (estrogen replacement therapy, prednisone, oral birth control pills, etc.) and have gained weight since starting the hormones, consult your doctor for the necessary adjustments.

19. If you have a health condition institute the HEALING DIET for the weight-loss phase. This diet creates a transition of your metabolism to fat-burning that will, in time, greatly diminish your hunger, while providing the essential nutrients needed for hearty

vitality and without creating a dangerous state of advanced ketosis.

20. If you started your diet with HEALING DIET foods, lose your final few pounds on the TRANSITIONAL DIET. Every thin person has developed the ability to lose a few pounds while eating normal foods, without skipping meals or instituting drastic measures. You too must acquire this skill.

21. If you are overweight but healthy you may select foods from THE DIET FOR THE REST OF YOUR LIFE for your weight loss plan.

22. Exercise for at least twenty minutes five times per week. As your weight drops, the amount of effort needed to exercise will decrease, making the exercise much more rewarding and enabling you to do more if you choose. Do not think of exercise as a fast way to lose weight. To lose one pound of fat, you must walk about thirty-five miles. Think of exercise as a way of increasing metabolism, normalizing your appetite, strengthening your heart—a way to create peace of mind, improve the quality of your sleep, and work off overindulgence or poor food choices.

23. Drink 1/2 oz of chlorine-free water for every pound of body weight daily as the symptoms of dehydration are easily confused with hunger.

24. Stop all carbonated beverages, both sugared and artificially sweetened and strictly limit your intake of sweet fruit drinks. Studies have shown that people who drink either artificially sweetened soft drinks or sweetened soft drinks daily are more likely to gain weight.

25. Do not think you can return to your old eating habits after you have met your goal. Use your version of the DIET FOR THE REST OF YOUR LIFE to maintain your weight.

26. At every opportunity, eat fish and their oils, olive oil, avocados, nuts and seeds, all the vegetable oils, and take as a supplement the essential fatty acid oils 2–4 grams a day, such as fish or flaxseed oil with borage seed oil. These are the things that your body craves.

27. High potency multiple vitamin, mineral and amino acid powder: 1 tbs daily. This will provide the essential amino acids, vitamins, minerals, and trace minerals necessary for robust vitality. If you do not use this type of supplement, these elements must be met by some other means.

28. Chromium picolinate: 400–800 micrograms daily.

29. Noni juice: 1/2 to 1 oz prior to meals and bedtime.

30. Coenzyme Q10/L-carnitine: 30 mg/250 mg 1-2 gel caps daily for cellular energy.

31. Glucomannan fiber: 575 mg 4-6 capsules daily with a large glass of water. Psyllium: 1 tbs in water daily is another fiber option.

32. Probiotics with fructo-oligosaccharides: 1-2 tablets daily during weight loss then 1-2 tablets weekly thereafter.

33. If you have any type of fungal disease, fungal toenails, jock itch, athletes foot, dandruff, or recurrent yeast infections, refer to the chapter on this subject to help you treat this problem. I think you will be amazed how much easier it is to lose weight when you are fungus free.

Richard L. Becker, .D.O.

NEVER LET A SURGEON BE THE ONLY ONE TO RECOMMEND AN ELECTIVE SURGERY . . . . IF YOU MADE $2,500 AN HOUR EVERY TIME YOU WALKED INTO AN OPERATING ROOM, YOU WOULD GO IN EVERY TIME YOU GOT THE CHANCE.

21

RECURRENT RESPIRATORY INFECTIONS AND THE COMMON COLD

Respiratory infections such as the common cold, earaches, streptococcal sore throat, sinusitis, bronchitis, and pneumonia are the most common diseases afflicting people of all ages. It is not unusual for a healthy person to come down with a cold, but it should resolve quickly, and they should have no more than a minor cold or two a year. For many, an increased frequency and severity of respiratory infections becomes an endless cycle of illness after illness, leading to multiple doctor visits and antibiotic use. The insult to the intestinal flora by repeated antibiotics and the chronic stress of being ill leads to a spiral of declining health, resulting in an open door to debilitating disease.

SOMETIMES, THE BEST REMEDY IS NO REMEDY AT ALL.

We, in America, have become a 7-Eleven society, unwilling to be inconvenienced by even a short wait. I, like everyone else, do not enjoy these colds. They can make you miserable for a week or more. It is tempting for both doctor and patient to start an antibiotic at the first sign of the sniffles. But I urge you to think twice before you do.

A few fundamental holistic concepts might help you form a viable plan to break the cycle of recurring respiratory infections. First, the majority of respiratory infections are viral and thus unresponsive to antibiotics. Second, even exposure once or twice a year to systemic broad-spectrum antibiotics can seriously disturb the natural intestinal bacterial flora, leading to severe consequences decades later. Yes, decades later. The intestinal tract's normal bacterial flora is one of our primary immune curtains of defense. The indiscriminate use of antibiotics can seriously compromise this vital immune function. And third, resorting to antibiotics too early in the course of even a bacterial respiratory infection can result in a diminished antibody response to the germ, thereby compromising your long-term immunity and leaving you prone to recurrent infections by similar germs in the future.

The propensity to develop an infection by any agent is governed by three basic principles: the virulence or disease-causing capability of the germ, the number of germs you are exposed to, and the disease-fighting immune potential of the host—you. Boosting the immune response of the host and decreasing the exposure to germs is the most effective way to restore health to those stuck in a cycle of recurrent respiratory infections.

Today's germs are supercharged antibiotic-resistant powerhouses, all too often capable of resisting the effect of the best antibiotic agents now being made. We must tilt this disease-causing equation in our favor by boosting immunity, improving hygiene and lifestyle traits, supplementing essential nutrients, and correcting altered bowel flora induced by antibiotics to restore vital health.

THE PRACTICE OF MEDICINE IS AN ART FORM. IF YOUR HEALTH PORTRAIT IS NOT TAKING SHAPE BY THE FOURTH DOCTOR VISIT, COMMISSION A NEW ARTIST.

We hear over and over about the development of antibiotic-resistant germs and the great difficulty in treating infections caused by them. America's pharmaceutical companies have tried to keep pace by making new and more powerful antibiotics. However, there is a limit even to their abilities and budgets. Eventually, drugs will be so powerful, toxic, and expensive no one will be able to afford them in any sense. Antibiotics have saved thousands of lives, and I am NOT telling you to never take them. If you become ill, and after forty-eight to seventy-two hours you continue to worsen, seek the help of your doctor, who can perform a simple blood test (complete blood count), throat culture, or quick streptococcal throat smear, which will help determine if you really need an antibiotic. If so, take the complete course as prescribed. While taking the antibiotic, and for two to four weeks after completing the course of treatment, strictly avoid sugar and starchy foods and restore the bowel's natural flora with the measures outlined below. This will help prevent a cycle of recurrent infections that can lead to serious health complications.

ALL MEDICATIONS HAVE SIDE EFFECTS, EVEN PLACEBOS.

Over the centuries, the human race has endured thousands of plagues and countless germs. Only the strong survived this relentless attack of infectious agents. This heritage is within you. Your ability to fight can be improved. Stick with it. With time and effort, your vital health can be restored!

Rx

RECOMMENDATIONS FOR RECURRENT RESPIRATORY INFECTIONS

1. If you have allergies, chronic sinusitis or asthma, they must be brought under control. If your home or work environment is contaminated with mold, this must be cleaned out. See the chapter on these conditions and incorporate the recommendations outlined into your program.

2. If you have any type of anemia, this must be corrected.

3. If you have a deficiency of ANY of the essential dietary elements, this must be corrected.

4. If you have, at any time in your life taken multiple rounds of antibiotics for any reason, or have been on an antibiotic for a prolonged period of time, for any reason, start the HEALING DIET and continue the diet until your health shows a pattern of vitality. Advance to the TRANSITIONAL DIET as tolerated and then to the DIET FOR THE REST OF YOUR LIFE.

5. If you have any condition that obstructs the flow of air through the nose, such as a deviated septum or

one that blocks the normal drainage of the sinuses, this must be addressed. It may require surgery.

6. Poor dental health is a major health risk. Brush and floss after every meal. Change your toothbrush every week until the cycle of infection is broken; then replace your toothbrush monthly.

7. Make every effort to improve your sleep quality. The immune system is most active during sleep.

8. Engage in gentle exercise for at least twenty minutes four times weekly. Exercise activates the immune system. As your health improves, increase the amount of exercise as tolerated.

9. Reduce the stress in your life. Chronic stress causes a release of hormones that inhibit the immune system. We all have times of stress that cannot be avoided, but long-term stress should be addressed and altered. For example, people who work the graveyard shift (11 p.m. – 7 a.m.) have been shown to have more frequent infections than people who work during the day and sleep at night.

10. Improve your hygiene practices. Frequent hand-washing and daily bathing decrease the transmission of germs. Never eat or drink using someone's glass or dish.

11. Drink 1/2 oz of chlorine-free water per pound of body weight daily. Ample hydration improves immunity. Dehydration suppresses immunity. By simply filtering your tap water with a charcoal filter, you can reduce your rate of colds and flu by up to 70 percent.

12. Vitamin C with bioflavonoids: 1–2 grams daily.

13. Zinc: 25–50 mg daily. Vitamin C and zinc may be used together during a cold as a lozenge and in pill form as a preventive measure. Commercially available zinc lozenges and nasal sprays are very effective in shortening the course of the common cold. If administered on a daily basis they are also effective in preventing colds.

14. Vitamin A and beta-carotene: 15,000 I.U. total daily. CAUTION: do not exceed 8,000 I.U. of vitamin A daily if you are pregnant or expect to conceive.

15. B-Complex: 50 mg up to 3 times daily.

16. Vitamin E: 400 I.U. daily.

17. Calcium: 1–2 grams daily, magnesium: 500–1,000 mg daily, and a source of trace minerals like sea kelp: 1–2 grams daily to provide the essential mineral selenium.

18. Essential amino acids: 2–3 grams daily.

19. High potency multiple vitamin, mineral and amino acid powder: 1 tbs daily may be used in place of numbers 12–18.

20. Fish or flaxseed oil with borage seed oil: 2 grams of each daily.

21. Noni juice: 1–4 oz daily on an empty stomach.

22. Quercetin: 500 mg daily.

23. Bee propolis: 500 mg daily. Bee Royal jelly: 100 mg daily. Bee pollen: 200 mg daily. There are combination products available that have similar amounts of the above ingredients. CAUTION: Do not take any bee products if you are allergic to bees.

24. Beta glucan: 10 mg 1 or 2 capsules daily.

25. Sinus-wash with grapefruit seed extract and oregano: 1-2 drops or puffs per nostril 1-2 times daily. This simple remedy is immensely helpful for colds that cause nasal congestion or aggravate chronic sinusitis. This type of sinus-wash is a wonderful natural antibiotic that will not disturb your intestinal

flora balance. You may open one capsule of beta glucan and pour the contents into the sinus wash for an excellent cold remedy.

26. Olive leaf extract: 100 mg twice daily.

27. Oil of oregano: 5 drops in water or 1 gel cap twice daily.

28. If your colds are accompanied with the herpes simplex virus or cold sores add L-lysine: 1 gram twice daily and apply oil of oregano: 1 drop directly onto cold sore 2-3 times daily.

29. Echinacea purpurea: 80 mg daily. May be used for as long as necessary to restore health.

30. Garlic both as a spice and a supplement: 3–5 grams daily.

31. Probiotics with fructo-oligosaccharides: 1-2 tablets daily on an empty stomach for at least 90 days to restore intestinal flora. You may supplement probiotics while taking prescription antibiotics. Taking them several hours apart will help assure maximum probiotic benefit. Once your health has improved, take a probiotic once or twice a week to help maintain your health.

32. Glucomannan fiber: 575 mg 4-6 capsules daily with a large glass of water. Psyllium: 1 tbs in water daily is another fiber option.

Richard L. Becker, .D.O.

HERBS AND VITAMINS SHOULD BE TREATED

WITH THE SAME RESPECT AS MEDICATIONS.

22

ACNE AND ROSACEA

The standard "peer-reviewed" science-based medical literature states that WHAT you eat has no bearing on the condition of acne and rosacea. After reading this book, if you now believe this statement to be true I have failed you miserably. How could ANY condition, syndrome, or disease NOT be affected by our diet? Does not the absence of food lead to death by starvation? And does not death by starvation include all parts of the human body, including the skin?

EVERY PERSON SHOULD HAVE A FAMILY PHYSICIAN OR GENERAL INTERNIST AS AN ADVOCATE. NEVER FORGET THAT AN ORGAN SPECIALIST HAS FORGOTTEN A LOT ABOUT THE OTHER ORGANS.

To say diet has no bearing in the treatment of acne or rosacea is to throw out every one of our life's experiences and volumes of accepted understandings in biochemistry, physiology, and nutrition-based pathology, along with the entire premise that the quality of our food affects our quality of life. I am not falling for it and neither should you. What you can conclude from this absurd statement is that all information concerning your health must be tempered with common sense, no matter the source.

Perhaps the most important point to be understood for the person who is battling acne or rosacea is that their skin condition may be the proverbial tip of the iceberg. Their skin is reflecting the body's misaligned control systems, and if not corrected, a serious health challenge eventually will follow.

To be successful in the treatment of acne and rosacea, one or more of the following physiologic aberrations must be addressed.

ABERRATIONS THAT MAY RESULT IN ACNE OR ROSACEA

1. Nutritional inadequacies

2. Reduced stomach acid and pancreatic secretions

3. Alterations in microbial flora of intestines and skin

4. Altered ability of skin bacteria and mites to turn skin oils into inflammatory oils

5. Plugging of skin pores by keratin

6. Hormone imbalance and fluctuations

7. Skin glucose elevation

8. Stress

9. Topical products that irritate the skin

10. Excoriation of the skin (picking)

The skin is an organ of excretion and elimination, as are the kidneys, lungs, liver, and intestinal tract. If the liver, kidneys, and intestines are out of balance, the skin is called upon to help with the normal process of elimination. The body's toxic waste material may be eliminated, in part, by the sweat glands. This creates a nutrient source for abnormal skin bacteria and mites. The intestinal bacteria sets the tone for the skin bacteria. Intestines hold a reserve of three to four pounds of microbes, and this flora is reflected on our skin. If the gut is off, the skin will be also. Many medications affect delicate intestinal bacterial flora, which play such an important role in our health and well-being. The primary culprits include antibiotics, hormones, and any medication that constipates, relieves pain, or suppresses stomach acid production.

Why then do so many doctors prescribe systemic antibiotics for the treatment of acne and rosacea? In the short term antibiotics can create a dramatic improvement of the skin and in the long term the skin doctors never treat the systemic complications induced by their therapies. But they should. It seems every day I see a patient who suffers from the conditions we have discussed in this book, and they all have taken either long-term antibiotics for acne and rosacea or have taken dozens of rounds of antibiotics for various infectious conditions. I urge you to exhaust every option available before you resort to systemic antibiotics in the treatment of acne and rosacea. There are times when taking an antibiotic for a year or longer is in your health's interest—when treating tuberculosis, for example—but not when the problem is acne or rosacea.

During adolescence, sex hormones may surge and create imbalances that promote acne. This phenomenon can continue well into mature adulthood. The hormone testosterone plays a role in acne and is the reason males have a higher occurrence of acne than females. However, excessive progesterone may also cause acne in women. This phenomenon has led many women to take oral contraceptives in an attempt to control acne. It is rarely necessary to take hormones to calm this imbalance. If the essential elements needed to manufacture and control hormones are present in the diet and supplements, most people can avoid such a drastic measure as hormone manipulation.

Stress plays a huge role in this hormone instability. When under stress, cortisol is released into the bloodstream. Cortisol is normal and essential to life, but excess cortisol is dangerous and plays a role in diseases associated with stress. Proper sleep, exercise, calcium, magnesium, zinc, vitamin A, and the essential B vitamins help in ways that no medication can in controlling the body's response to stress.

It has been my observation that individuals with severe acne often have deficiencies in these nutrients and typically will respond dramatically, over time, when these elements are replaced. Megadoses are not necessary, and I do not recommend them without the direct involvement of a physician experienced in these matters. We also know that a deficiency in chromium can result in elevated blood sugar, and that chromium is deficient in the typical American diet. Studies of acne patients' skin have shown an elevation of glucose

IN THE SKIN that returns to normal when trace amounts of chromium are supplemented.

Rosacea affects more women than men and usually occurs in middle age and beyond, but it can affect twenty-year-olds. Rosacea has been associated with the colonization of the skin by a skin mite called *Demodex folliculorum*. It is of interest to note that laboratory rats can be successfully inoculated with this skin mite only if they are deficient in the essential B vitamin, riboflavin. Riboflavin is found in abundance in green leafy vegetables, meats, and whole grains. Deficiencies of riboflavin are most likely to occur in those who ingest a refined grain and processed diet or those who are taking oral contraceptives or multiple medications. It has been my experience that rosacea responds well to B vitamin replacement. Rosacea has also been found to be associated with a reduced secretion of stomach acid and pancreatic enzymes. Both conditions are remediable with proper supplementation.

It is important for those who suffer from either acne or rosacea to be careful about what comes in contact with their skin. Many cosmetic products can aggravate their condition. Look for the term noncomedogenic when purchasing these agents, as these products usually do not cause flare-ups of delicate skin conditions.

Finally, you must understand that you cannot scrub or pick away acne and rosacea. However, good hygiene is essential. A gentle exfoliating skin cleanser removes old dead skin that may plug the skin pores. The skin is in a constant state of renewal. Plugs of dead skin can block the skin's pores and must be removed twice daily with gentle cleansing.

The same peer-reviewed medical standard we spoke of earlier makes a distinction between many conditions that look like acne and rosacea, such as excorea, folliculitis, keratosis pilaris, seborrhea, and others. Certainly these conditions have differences when compared to acne and rosacea, but their treatment is fundamentally the same. Do I need to explain why?

Rx

RECOMMENDATIONS FOR BOTH ACNE AND ROSACEA-LIKE SKIN CONDITIONS

1. If you have taken multiple rounds of antibiotics for any reason or have been on antibiotics for a prolonged period of time, for best results you must follow the HEALING DIET to correct intestinal dysbiosis. Be prepared for an initial flare of either acne or rosacea. After six to eight weeks the

flare will begin to calm for most. Advance to the TRANSITIONAL DIET as tolerated then onto the DIET FOR THE REST OF YOUR LIFE.

2. If you do not require the HEALING DIET, your diet must at least be free of sugar, refined grains, hydrogenated vegetable oils such as margarine, and processed foods as provided by the DIET FOR THE REST OF YOUR LIFE.

3. For every pound of body weight, drink 1/2 oz of chlorine-free water daily.

4. Milk thistle: 140 mg twice daily to improve liver function.

5. Glycolic cleanser, pH balanced: Use twice daily for gentle cleansing of the affected skin areas.

6. Calendula officinalis (marigold) and Hypericum perforatum (St. John's wort) botanical toner: Apply this herbal formula to freshly cleansed skin twice daily to help reduce the skin's abnormal microbes.

7. Tea tree oil: Apply sparingly to areas of skin inflammation and acne sores twice daily after cleansing and toning.

8. Olive leaf extract: 100 mg twice daily for yeast suppression.

9. Oil of oregano: 2-5 drops in water 1-2 times daily. Oil of oregano can be applied directly on affected skin at bedtime.

10. Oil of primrose: 1–2 grams daily by mouth. If this amount makes your skin too oily, decrease to your comfort level.

11. Probiotics with fructo-oligosaccharides: 1-2 tablets on an empty stomach daily until skin has greatly improved; then take 1 or 2 doses a week to maintain healthy skin.

12. Glucomannan fiber: 575 mg 4-6 capsules daily with a large glass of water. Psyllium: 1 tbs in water daily is another fiber option.

13. High potency multiple vitamin, mineral and amino acid powder: 1 tbs daily in water.

14. Natural source vitamin A: 50,000 I.U. daily for 30 days followed by 25,000 I.U. daily for 30 days, then use a high potency multiple vitamin, mineral and amino acid powder for your vitamin A source

of 8,500 I.U. daily thereafter. If you find taking extra vitamin A with the vitamin powder helps to maintain healthy skin, you may do so safely as long as it is a natural source vitamin A and the total daily dose of vitamin A is under 25,000 I.U. CAUTION: do not take more than 8,000 I.U. of vitamin A if you are pregnant or may become pregnant.

15. Noni juice: 1 oz twice daily. Many people have found it helpful to apply Noni juice directly onto the skin at bedtime.

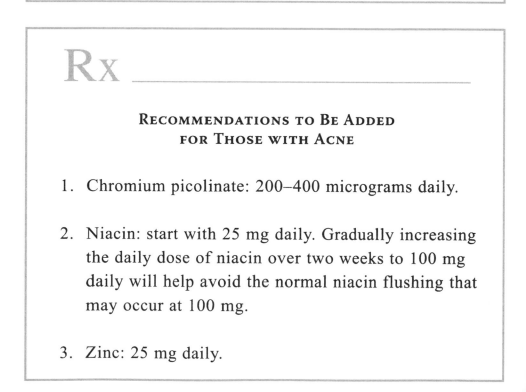

Rx

RECOMMENDATIONS TO BE ADDED FOR THOSE WITH ACNE

1. Chromium picolinate: 200–400 micrograms daily.

2. Niacin: start with 25 mg daily. Gradually increasing the daily dose of niacin over two weeks to 100 mg daily will help avoid the normal niacin flushing that may occur at 100 mg.

3. Zinc: 25 mg daily.

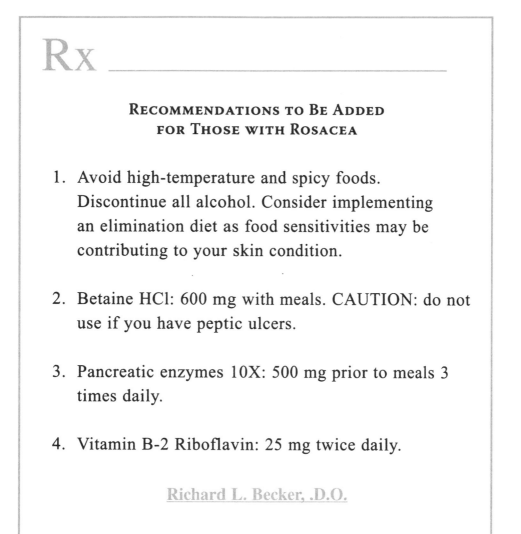

Rx

RECOMMENDATIONS TO BE ADDED
FOR THOSE WITH ROSACEA

1. Avoid high-temperature and spicy foods. Discontinue all alcohol. Consider implementing an elimination diet as food sensitivities may be contributing to your skin condition.

2. Betaine HCl: 600 mg with meals. CAUTION: do not use if you have peptic ulcers.

3. Pancreatic enzymes 10X: 500 mg prior to meals 3 times daily.

4. Vitamin B-2 Riboflavin: 25 mg twice daily.

Richard L. Becker, .D.O.

AFTER A GOOD PHARMACIST, THE NEXT BEST FRIEND IS A KNOWLEDGEABLE HEALTH FOOD STORE ATTENDANT.

23

IRRITABLE BOWEL SYNDROME
a disease or another example of
INTESTINAL DYSBIOSIS AND CANDIDIASIS

The most common chronic intestinal complaint in America for which the advice of a doctor is sought is irritable bowel syndrome (IBS). The person who suffers from this painful condition has abdominal bloating, constipation frequently alternating with loose stool, and at times intense spasms of the intestinal tract. One in five Americans has this syndrome, and most are women. If the problem is severe enough, the frustrated patient will eventually receive a full gastrointestinal work-up, including scans, barium-enhanced X rays, and intestinal endoscopy. Then, she will be told by her doctor that no signs of disease could be found, and that the patient has a nervous or spastic intestinal tract, for which there is no cure.

One cannot help but wonder if irritable bowel syndrome is a disease caused by faulty genetics we do not understand or by a heretofore-unknown germ; or, is it just another example of imbalances in the intestinal microflora known as intestinal dysbiosis?

I am again reminded of Harry Truman's statement, "The only thing new is the history you don't know." In 1908, Dr. Elie Metchnikoff, received a Nobel Prize for recognizing and clarifying the critical link between the delicate balance of microbial life forms in the intestinal tract and a long vigorous life. (See Chapter 4—THE BEGINNING TO THE END.)

Dr. Metchnikoff taught us nearly 100 years ago that a typical healthy adult has approximately three pounds of bacteria, yeast, protozoa, and amoeba of varying types in their intestinal tract. He showed us that half of the stool's weight is from these normally occurring life forms. These organisms serve numerous vital functions. They help to digest foods. They make essential vitamins such as cyanocobalamine (vitamin B-12) and vitamin K. They perform a critical role in the body's immune response in the constant battle with infecting organisms, such as shigella, salmonella, and the ongoing battle with cancer we all face, not only in the intestinal tract but in all our physiologic systems.

Further scientific discoveries have shown us that a healthy intestinal tract requires certain key elements. Every one of the essential vitamins, minerals, trace minerals, fatty acids, and amino acids must be present—not just at the minimal daily requirement levels but with a little extra left over to provide for your uniqueness or for times of stress. The food ingested must be a balanced blend of whole foods, each meal complete in its nutrients. There must be raw, fresh fruits, and vegetables with high levels of fiber. Also, there must be a daily dietary source of the beneficial microorganisms that colonize our intestinal tract. This is achieved by eating a diet with fresh, raw garden vegetables, whole grain foods, complete with fermented items such as yogurt, buttermilk, sauerkraut, cottage cheese, and sour cream, just as our ancestors have for thousands of years.

Although the physiology and science of the intestinal tract is complicated, the lifestyle practices that lead to healthy intestines and thus robust vitality are not. If the food has been refined, altered, overly preserved, sugared, fortified, pre-packaged, salted, or processed do not make this type of food a daily source of nutrients. An occasional treat is allowed, of course, and there will be times (while traveling, for example) when your choices are limited, but these "fast foods" cannot be the foundation of your diet, as so many of us have made them today.

If the diet is suboptimal, infectious disease invariably results, often requiring systemic antibiotics. These medications, although potentially lifesaving, ALWAYS affect the normal intestinal microbes, as well as the infecting germs. If healthy lifestyle measures are in place, the system is perfectly capable of "resetting" itself with just a few simple measures. If the antibiotics are taken for long periods of time, taken with immune-suppressive medications such as steroids, or taken with a refined, high-sugar diet, dire consequences are inevitable.

One of the most serious consequences of this scenario is the infestation of the intestinal tract with disease-causing strains of yeast and fungi. There are tens of thousands of different fungi, and hundreds are known to cause disease. Occurring as microbes, the fungi are most complex. In the grand scheme of nature, fungi fill the recycling roll. If a tree falls in the forest, it is the fungi that reduce the wood to its basic elements so that the next tree can grow. If a forest animal dies, this same recycling process releases nutrients to provide for the next generation of life. Some of these fungal organisms have developed the ability to hasten the process of recycling by poisoning (with mycotoxins) those who may ingest or become infected by them. We have all heard of unfortunate people who have died after ingesting poisonous mushrooms. This is uncommon and a fate that is easy to avoid. What is strikingly common is the growth of this type of organism in the intestinal tract. Virtually every breath of air we breathe has fungal spores in it. Every bite of fresh fruit and vegetables has yeast and mold spores on its peel. This is normal. If the intestinal microflora have been altered, as in intestinal dysbiosis, normal inhibition of fungal proliferation is suboptimal, resulting in disease states —either by infection, the release of fungal toxins, or both.

If the intestinal flora is altered, the microflora of skin, hair, nails, and genitalia eventually will be altered as well. Seborrhea, dandruff, fungal toenails, vaginal yeast infections, ringworm, jock itch, and athlete's foot are all caused by fungi or yeast. These conditions are notoriously difficult to treat, often requiring prolonged use of medications simply to keep them from becoming worse, the sufferer having long ago given up hope for a cure. The key to the cure is in the intestines and the realignment achieved by the HEALING DIET and the measures listed below.

If you have been suffering from virtually any condition, from allergies to seborrhea, even cancer, and you have not addressed ANY coexisting form of a fungal disease, you will not make optimal progress. The scope of this text does not allow for complete discussion of this topic, but be advised that modern science has shown that the lowly mold is capable of causing great misery, including your health challenges.

If Dr. Metchnikoff were alive today, I think he would receive another Nobel Prize for his work in curing irritable bowel syndrome.

Rx _____

RECOMMENDATIONS FOR IRRITABLE BOWEL SYNDROME

1. First, see your doctor for an accurate diagnosis. IBS is very common and not life-threatening; however it may be easily confused with more serious medical conditions such as Crohn's disease and ulcerative colitis.

2. If you have taken multiple rounds of antibiotics for any reason or have taken antibiotics for a prolonged period of time, received steroid therapy (prednisone etc.), hormone replacement therapy, or oral birth control pills at any time in your life, follow the HEALING DIET until your pattern of well-being returns, and then follow the TRANSITIONAL DIET. Upon the implementation of the TRANSITIONAL DIET if your health declines, return to the HEALING DIET. Eventually you should be able to progress to the DIET FOR THE REST OF YOUR LIFE. This entire process may take up to three years for some.

3. Whether you require the HEALING DIET or not, strictly avoid sorbitol, mannitol, lactose, corn syrup, fructose as an added sweetener (the low amounts of fructose in the HEALING DIET fruits are permissible), artificial sweeteners, carbonated beverages, sugar, and all dairy products except those allowed on the HEALING DIET. You will have better success if you minimize your grain intake, especially wheat and all its derived products.

4. Increase your fiber intake from raw fruits and vegetables and avoid fiber derived from grains such as wheat bran as most IBS sufferers are intolerant of grain fiber.

5. Dramatically reduce your caffeine intake and increase your chlorine-free water intake.

6. Consider implementing an elimination diet or eat for your blood type. Approximately seventy percent of all IBS sufferers have developed some type of food sensitivities that can be controlled by avoiding those foods that induce immune reactions.

7. Limit starch intake (beans and grains) and emphasize protein and essential fatty acid (olive oil, etc.) intake.

8. In order to succeed in the management of IBS, stress levels must be reduced. Exercise, spirituality, and proper sleep manage stress like no medication can. Also, biofeedback can help stop the recurrent cycle of stress-induced intestinal illness.

9. Carefully review all the medications you take whether prescribed or over the counter for intestinal side effects, as they may be contributing to your complaints.

10. Glucomannan fiber: 575 mg 3-9 capsules daily with a large glass of water. This soluble fiber source is remarkably well tolerated. Psyllium: 1 tbs in water daily is another fiber option however it is not as well tolerated.

11. Probiotics with fructo-oligosaccharides: 1 tablet daily for at least six months then 1-2 tablets a week thereafter.

12. Fish or flaxseed oil with borage seed oil: 2 grams of each daily.

13. Milk thistle: 300 mg daily.

14. Enteric-coated delayed-release oil of peppermint:

90 mg twice daily on an empty stomach. Oil of peppermint must be enteric-coated, or it may cause stomach and esophagus irritation.

15. High potency multiple vitamin, mineral and amino acid powder: 1 tbs daily.

16. Noni juice: 1–2 oz daily.

17. If there is any evidence of a fungal infection such as athlete's foot, jock itch, seborrhea, tinea versicolor, or recurrent vaginal yeast infections, refer to Chapter 25 on this subject and include the anti-fungal measures in your plan.

Richard L. Becker, .D.O.

24

O S T E O P O R O S I S

Osteoporosis is a bone disease that causes a decrease of bone mass, resulting in thin, weak bones susceptible to fracture. This is common knowledge today, but what you may not know is that osteoporosis is a painful condition that may result from a multitude of reasons over a long period of time.

EACH AND EVERY ONE OF US CARRIES THE ULTIMATE RESPONSIBILITY OF OUR HEALTH CARE CHOICES.

Bodies assimilate bone mass steadily until the age of thirty-five. After thirty-five, it is normal to slowly lose bone strength, but the rate of loss should be slow. In a normal setting, the accumulation of bone early in life is more than enough to last a lifetime. Unfortunately, some people lose bone at an accelerated rate, leaving them susceptible to pain, declining stature, and multiple bone fractures. There are over ten million Americans who suffer from osteoporosis and two million of them are men. There are also thirty-four million Americans with low bone mass placing them at increased risk for future osteoporosis.

We are told daily to drink more milk in an effort to build strong bones. In America we consume more dairy products than any other country, yet we have the highest rate of osteoporosis worldwide. Clearly, drinking milk is not the answer in preventing osteoporosis.

Due to the potential disastrous effects of this disabling and painful condition, the media and the pharmaceutical industry have created near mass hysteria in an effort to create a market for the drugs approved for the prevention and treatment of thin fragile bones.

Do we all need to take a medication for osteoporosis? Do we all need an expensive and potentially toxic tonic that in reality can only slow the rate of bone loss?

I am asked on a daily basis, "My DEXA bone scan shows loss of bone. Shouldn't I be taking something for it?" Some do need the medication, but who?

Many medications are now on the market for the treatment and prevention of osteoporosis, including Fosamax, Didronel, Miacalcin, Nolvadex, Evista, all the estrogen products, and many more to come. Just a few moments spent with a *Physicians' Desk Reference* reading about the potential side effects of these medications is enough to create panic, even in the mind of a seasoned physician. How can anyone expect to come to a rational decision about the path to take in the treatment and prevention of osteoporosis?

It is the ultimate responsibility of each of us to make the decision about what medications to take. The days of the doctor making all our choices are over. Blind trust is not in the patient's best interest. There are certainly times when we cannot make such decisions—in emergency, surgical, or intensive care settings, for example—but the management of osteoporosis is not one of these.

Let's talk a little medical common sense to help you make this important decision. The first concept to understand is that osteoporosis does not attack one day out of the blue with no warning! It is a lifetime in the making. The progression of osteoporosis is influenced by many normal physiological principles and risk factors, just as cancer is influenced by many variables. Lung cancer is relatively common in smokers but rare among those who do not smoke. Such is the case with osteoporosis. Understanding the risk factors and body functions will help you to make a sound decision.

Accumulation of bone mass when young and slowing its loss while aging are the critical factors in preventing the disease of osteoporosis. How strong the bones become and/or eventually how weak they become is influenced by genetics, the amount of exercise stress we place on the bones, lifestyle factors, nutrition, coexisting disease, and normal hormone support of the bones.

Science recognizes that hormones play a critical role in bone strength, and this has led to many products now available to treat osteoporosis. It has been proven beyond any doubt that normal levels of estrogen, testosterone, and progesterone maintain bone mass. It has also been proven beyond doubt that these hormones, when given in excess, can do great harm, including weight gain, hypertension, cancer, and much more.

The controversy and mixed information surrounding hormone replacement therapy and the prevention and treatment of osteoporosis is enough to terrify any thinking person. Where in this storm of confusion is a safe harbor?

A clear understanding of the known risk factors for osteoporosis is the key to understanding who should take what medications.

Osteoporosis is not caused by a pathogen, such as a bacteria or virus; it is the result of many influences. I have listed below the known risk factors for osteoporosis. Read through the list and make a mark by

A FEW MOMENTS READING A *PHYSICIANS' DESK REFERENCE* PRIOR TO TAKING A MEDICATION MAY CHANGE YOUR MIND.

each of the risk factors you have, and then total the score. Your score will help you make a sound decision—one that could prevent much suffering and expense in your life.

RISK FACTORS FOR OSTEOPOROSIS

1. Female gender

2. Caucasian or Asian ancestry

3. Family history of osteoporosis

4. Slight bone structure with thin body type

5. Bone density T-score greater than one

6. Prolonged bed rest greater than one month

7. Long-term smoking

8. Long-term alcohol use

9. Malnourishment

10. Diet low in minerals, especially calcium

11. High dairy intake with a low intake of fruits and vegetables

12. Diets high in sugar and salt

13. Drinking more than two cups of coffee daily

14. High carbonated beverage intake

15. Extremely high protein and meat diet

16. Sedentary lifestyle

17. History of cancer and chemotherapy

18. Chronic liver disease

19. Chronic kidney disease

20. Long-term use of seizure medication

21. Steroid therapy for longer than two months (prednisone, dexamethasone, strong topical steroids, etc.)

22. Long-term use of heparin

23. Hyperthyroidism, hyperparathyroidism or any endocrine disorder

24. Early menopause prior to age forty with no hormone replacement therapy or soy and wild yam extract supplementation

25. Hysterectomy with ovary removal prior to age forty with no hormone replacement therapy or soy and wild yam supplementation

26. Never have given birth to a child

27. Reduced sun exposure, such as from long-term office work

28. Vitamin D deficiency

29. Testosterone deficiency

30. Any type of intestinal condition that may affect the body's ability to absorb nutrients, such as Crohn's

disease, ulcerative colitis, stomach bypass surgery or partial removal of any part of the intestines. (This does not include irritable bowel syndrome.)

How was your score?

If you have 0–3 marks, forget about osteoporosis. Just continue to live the good life you have been living.

If you have 4–6 marks, you need lifestyle changes, vitamins, minerals, safe plant-extract hormone support when appropriate (see Chapter 18 for menopause management), a wholesome diet, and exercise, not drug therapy.

OSTEOPOROSIS IS BONE DISEASE A LIFETIME IN THE MAKING.

If you have 7–9 marks, you need maximum protection with intensive nutritional support, vitamins, maximum safe mineral supplementation, gentle exercise, and bio-identical hormone replacement therapy, when appropriate, to slow down your bone loss.

If you have ten or more marks, you need the help of an expert in the management of your inevitable thin bones, including lifestyle changes, intensive dietary measures, maximum safe mineral supplementation, bone forming supplements, bio-identical hormone replacement therapy, and osteoporosis medication.

If you are under thirty-five years of age, and have a high score, you can reverse the trend toward osteoporosis. Take this as an early warning and make a change for the better. Those of you over thirty-five should consider that it is never too late to improve your health. Make the list of recommendations below a part of your life. Your bones will thank you for the change!

Rx

RECOMMENDATIONS FOR OSTEOPOROSIS TREATMENT AND PREVENTION

1. Multiple mineral: containing calcium up to 2 grams, magnesium up to 1 gram, boron 3 mg, copper 3 mg, zinc 25 mg, manganese 2 mg, vitamin D 400 I.U. vitamin K 80 micro-grams daily and a source of trace minerals such as sea kelp 1 gram daily.

2. B-complex: 100 mg daily.

3. Vitamin A: 5,000 I.U. daily.

4. Vitamin C: 1 gram daily.

5. Vitamin E: 400 I.U. daily.

6. Essential amino acids: 1 tbs daily.

7. High potency multiple vitamin, mineral and amino acid powder: 1 tbs daily may be substituted for numbers 1–6. If your osteoporosis score is over 7, you will need to add an extra source of minerals such as microcrystalline hydroxyapatite (bone meal) to the high potency multiple in order to attain maximal safe mineral intake.

8. Glucosamine sulfate: 300 mg up to 5 tablets daily.

9. Chondroitin sulfate: 200 mg up to 5 tablets daily.

10. Methylsulfonylmethane (MSM): 300 mg up to 5 tablets daily.

11. Fish or flaxseed oil with borage seed oil: 2 grams of each daily.

12. Eat less dairy, red meat, sugar, and salt.

13. Eat more soy, green leafy vegetables, broccoli, beans, nuts and seeds, eggs, onion, garlic, whole grains, sardines, flounder, and salmon for calcium and bone-forming nutrients.

14. Eliminate all carbonated beverages from your diet.

15. Drink less coffee and consider switching to tea.

16. Follow a program of frequent, gentle, weight-bearing exercise.

17. Refer to Chapter 19—MENOPAUSE MANAGEMENT THE NATURAL WAY for safe plant-extract hormone support, and incorporate these measures into your plan for the management and prevention of osteoporosis.

Richard L. Becker, .D.O.

A LITTLE EXERCISE GOES A LONG WAY IN THE

PREVENTION OF DISEASE AND HUMAN SUFFERING.

25

FUNGI, YEAST, AND CANDIDA

old, mildew, yeast, fungi, and candida surround us. Virtually every breath you take carries mold spores. Thousands of fungal species inhabit the soil and are underfoot with every step. Candida and various fungal species are normal inhabitants of human skin, the intestinal tract, and mucous membranes. These organisms play a major role in nature's mechanism of recycling and decay.

When a human dies, the ubiquitous presence of these organisms allows for quick and efficient decomposition of the remains. For a vitally healthy person, fungi pose little or no threat. An optimally functioning immune system will actively seek out any invaders and destroy them. However, for the compromised person, the ever-present fungi and yeast may proliferate, creating an infection leading to a baffling syndrome of failing health.

There are thousands of fungal species, and at least 300 of them have been shown to cause disease in humans. Many times the disease process is slow and deceptively innocuous, creating an attitude of acceptance. Years may pass while the victim of nature's recycling fungal agents tolerates the annoyance of chronic sinusitis, jock itch, athlete's foot, fungal toenails, dandruff, or recurrent yeast infections, all the while unaware of fungi's ability to create poisonous mycotoxins. Alcohol is the most widely recognized fungal toxin, and we are all familiar with its potential toxic nature. However, there are thousands of these toxins, and they have been implicated as a cause of cancer, heart disease, arthritis, asthma, depression, and many more difficult-to-cure diseases.

If the person with athlete's foot, for example, has poor dietary habits, has taken multiple rounds of antibiotics, hormone replacement therapy, or prolonged courses of steroids, this person's natural barriers to infection may have become compromised. In addition, other disease causing fungi may colonize the airways leading to pneumonia. The intestinal tract may also become colonized, leading to the altered state of bowel flora called intestinal dysbiosis. If lifestyle and medication changes are not made, compromised immunity develops, and these opportunistic fungal organisms can gain access to vital organs through the circulatory system, creating a life-threatening disease.

Harrison's Principles of Internal Medicine is a standard text for most American medical schools. The text contains over twenty-five hundred pages of detailed descriptions of the signs, causes, mechanism, and treatment of human diseases. If the serious student manages to read and comprehend this seemingly inclusive text, she may be left with a false sense of security, since *Harrison's* dedicates only fourteen pages to the commonly recognized fungal diseases. It has been my experience that 40 percent of my patients have some type of fungal disorder, which complicates or causes their decline in health. Clearly, we need more research and understanding in this area.

You, however, do not need to wait for the medical community to catch up. Check the risk factors for fungal disease listed below. If your health has been failing and you have several of these factors in your history, you may now have the key to recovery. If your health is good, but you have more than a few of these factors, make some changes now to avoid the inevitable decline in health that awaits you.

RISK FACTORS FOR FUNGAL DISEASE

1. Prolonged antibiotic therapy for any reason, even if you took the medication many years ago

2. Short-term antibiotics taken frequently (even one round of antibiotics can cause athlete's foot or candida vaginitis)

3. Steroid therapy (prednisone, dexamethasone, etc., including steroid nasal sprays for the treatment of allergies and strong topical steroids for skin conditions, such as psoriasis or eczema)

4. Cancer

5. Chemotherapy

6. Radiation therapy

7. Oral birth control pills

8. Hormone replacement therapy

9. Malnourishment

10. Diets high in refined sugar and refined flour

11. Medications that constipate

12. Human immune virus with acquired immune deficiency syndrome

13. Long-term emotional or physical stress

14. Overwhelming environmental exposure to fungal spores and mold such as occurs after the flooding of a home

15. Poorly controlled diabetes

16. Pregnancy

17. Troublesome allergies well into adulthood

18. Travel to areas that harbor fungal spores, such as the American southwestern desert and Ohio River valley

19. Diets devoid of raw fruits, vegetables, and fermented foods such as yogurt, thereby altering beneficial bowel flora

20. Frequent consumption of moldy foods

21. High alcohol intake, especially active yeast-containing beverages, such as beer

22. Skin or intestinal barrier compromise such as occurs with intestinal flu-like viruses or skin rashes

23. Multiple sex partners or sexual partner with fungal disease

24. Exposure to contaminated shower and bathing surfaces as occurs in saunas and gyms

25. Never being breast-fed as an infant

26. Recurrent oral thrush or candida diaper rash as a baby

As you set out to make changes, keep in mind that to successfully cure a fungal disorder you must be persistent and complete in your treatment. Treatment only with medication, while lifestyle and nutritional changes are ignored, is short-sighted and doomed to fail. Holism is the key to success. Consider the list of recommendations below to guide you on your road to recovery. These recommendations have helped many regain their strong vitality.

Rx

RECOMMENDATIONS FOR FUNGAL DISEASE TREATMENT

1. If you are in failing health and have multiple risk factors or have been diagnosed with a fungal disease, follow the HEALING DIET until your pattern of vitality has been restored. Be prepared for a significant healing crisis. If you have gained weight, follow the HEALING DIET until your weight has normalized. To avoid unnecessary stress, lose the weight slowly. Advance to the TRANSITIONAL DIET as tolerated and then on to the DIET FOR THE REST OF YOUR LIFE. The complete dietary progression and treatment may take up to three years. This may seem dramatic and unattainable; however, most find they feel better and are more than willing to make permanent changes for better health.

2. High potency multiple vitamin, mineral and amino acid powder: 1 tbs. daily.

3. Glucomannan fiber: 575 mg 3-9 capsules daily with a large glass of water. This soluble fiber source is remarkably well tolerated. Psyllium: 1 tbs in water daily is another fiber option.

4. Probiotics: 1-2 tablets daily for at least six months then 1 tablet twice weekly thereafter.

5. Noni juice: 1–4 oz daily on an empty stomach.

6. Drink 1/2 oz chlorine-free water per pound of body weight daily.

7. Beta glucan: 10 mg twice daily.

8. There are many naturally occurring antiyeast and fungal herbs and food extracts available today. The following is a list you will find helpful. Not everyone will need to take all of these agents. Most find cycling through several of them helpful, being on two or three at a time. It is usually obvious to the person which remedies help the most.

   a. Garlic: 3–5 grams orally daily. Garlic can also be freshly cut and applied to any area of the skin or nails affected by fungus.

   b. Pau d'arco: 500–1,000 mg twice daily.

   c. Olive leaf extract: 100–200 mg twice daily.

   d. Caprylic acid: 500–1,000 mg twice daily.

e. Oil of oregano: 5–10 drops in water once or twice daily or 1 gel cap once or twice daily.

f. Unpasteurized apple cider vinegar: 1 tsp in water twice daily.

g. Tea tree oil: applied topically to fungal infected toenails daily for as long as eighteen months. The duration of treatment must allow enough time for the diseased nail to be replaced by a normal nail.

h. Vick's VapoRub: Vick's contains oil of eucalyptus, menthol, and camphor. It may be mixed with Tea tree oil and applied to fungal toenails daily with surprising effectiveness. Oil of oregano may also be used alone or in combination with Vick's VapoRub. The treatment must be continued for up to eighteen months so that a healthy nail may replace the infected nail.

i. Sinus-wash with grapefruit seed extract and oregano: 1-2 drops or puffs per nostril 1-2 times daily. This type of sinus-wash is a wonderful natural antifungal that has no systemic side effects. You may open one capsule of beta glucan and pour the contents into the sinus wash for immune system activation.

9. Complement your treatment of fungal disease with the recommendations listed for your coexisting health disorder as outlined in the chapters pertaining to your health issues.

10. Consider talking to your doctor about taking a prescriptive antifungal medication. Medications alone cannot be relied upon for a complete cure without the above holistic measures.

Richard L. Becker, .D.O.

26

A Foundation for Prevention

Holistic medicine is a catchphrase today. It has become a sound bite for the health food and vitamin industry, but what does it really mean? The obvious answer is to treat the entire body, not just an organ. This response is what we expect to hear.

THE BEST TREATMENT OF DISEASE IS PREVENTION .... IF YOU KNEW WHAT THE DOCTOR KNOWS, YOU WOULD USE MEDICATIONS ONLY AS A LAST RESORT.

There is more, much more to include in the definition of holistic medicine. If we are to change our health care system and our personal health for the better, we must include HOW to treat all our physiologic systems in concert. It will be difficult for the health care system to change because it is deeply entrenched in organ subspecialist and crisis intervention care. We as patients must change the way we think and this in time will spur change in the overall system. Throughout history change has always come from the people.

Although there are many references to prevention in medical literature today, they almost always refer to immunizations and health-screening tests, such as mammography for breast cancer and prostate specific antigen for prostate cancer. These tests do nothing to prevent or treat disease, and the number of immunizations a child must take today is staggering. Furthermore, it may be that some of them are not in the child's best interest. This is not my idea of holistic preventive medicine. Surely there is more we can do to prevent the suffering of our American citizens.

To understand the difference between holistic prevention and our current system of crisis intervention and medication-induced stalling of disease, consider the diagram and its explanation on the following page.

A mother, at her expense, provides all of the nutrition for a developing fetus in the womb. It is in the interest of the species that their progeny have this advantage. This kick-start to life is a huge plus. If even minimally acceptable nutrition follows for these children, they will grow to an

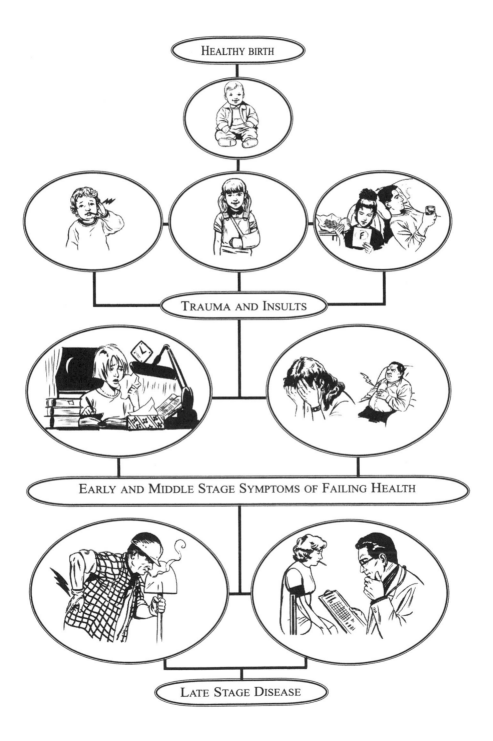

age when they, too, can reproduce. Again, this is in the best interest of the species.

As the boost in nutritional elements provided by a mother begins to subside and proper dietary intake of these elements is established, all is generally fine with just an occasional need of intervention for the youngster. This benefit to the child is obvious in that the leading cause of death in the one- to eighteen-year age group is accidental deaths, not diseases, such as heart disease and cancer in the mature person. The young also are generally not plagued by chronic afflictions commonly suffered by adults, such as arthritis, hypertension, and chronic fatigue. We think of the young as having all the advantages of youth—energy, vitality, and strength. These characteristics are not necessarily what keep a person alive in the modern world. Wisdom, precaution, experience, and the ability to work are far more valuable for survival. Yet the young thrive in spite of their lack of life skills.

If a child does not establish wholesome habits early in life, problems inevitably arise later in childhood or well into adulthood. The vitamin, mineral, protein, and essential fatty acid levels, along with an altered balance of the delicate intestinal flora of an individual, may drop below ideal, allowing minor aberrations in the system. This may not seem like much, but it gives the disease processes a foothold early in the life of a child. Initially, the problems are minor and easy to fix. But if a major insult occurs, such as pneumonia, long-term antibiotic therapy, hormone manipulation, or a major injury such as a motor vehicle accident, the decline in health may be greatly accelerated. With each successive drop in essential nutritional factors, there is an increase in disease potential and vague symptoms, represented by the steps in the diagram. Eventually, if left unchecked, a syndrome of dysfunction, characterized by multi-system complaints, unexplained by laboratory and x-ray diagnostic tests will follow, such as chronic fatigue, essential hypertension, and fibromyalgia.

The initiation and progression of most chronic health conditions follow a series of events as outlined above that eventually end in an incurable disease. It is the method of the pharmaceutical industry to know as many of the various biochemical steps as possible in this disease progression so that a patentable drug may be developed to stall the progression or relieve the symptoms of the syndrome but rarely to cure it. Hypertension is a perfect example of this concept. Blood-pressure drugs control hypertension but never cure it. The drug company now has a dependent customer for life.

Superior genetics certainly plays a role for those who are spared chronic disease, but the less fortunate cannot change what they have inherited. Eventually, when we can achieve genetic improvement, it is my opinion that we will find that genetic influences have less to do with a long healthy life than currently expected. If our genetics were primarily to blame, these bad genes would attract attention early in life as they do with most of currently known genetic diseases.

What must change is our fundamental approach to the treatment of chronically developing diseases. This change must start in utero (in the womb) by mothers for maximum effect. It can be instituted at any time in life as long as a patient is motivated and capable of change.

It is nutritional and lifestyle choices that make the biggest impact on vitality over time. If bad nutritional and lifestyle habits are established early in a child's life, there will be an inevitable price to pay. The price is a syndrome of chronic disease that has its base in nutritional deficiencies.

The reason so many chronic health conditions are considered incurable by current pharmaceutical methods is that underlying nutritional disorders are not being addressed early in life. The typical child has taken at least a dozen rounds of antibiotics by the time he reaches eighteen years of age. Though necessary at times, these courses of treatment set the stage for an imbalance of intestinal microbial flora, which ultimately affects our ability to heal, process nutrients, and maintain immunity.

This imbalance is easy to restore in childhood with simple avoidance of sugar and the administration of acidophilus and other methods of sustaining the intestinal flora during and after the use of antibiotics.

Most small children love sugar and will eat it at every opportunity. They rarely enjoy vegetables and will refuse these offerings repeatedly. They favor fatty and starchy foods and will request them in place of what an adult would consider wholesome. Their growth requires a higher level of essential fatty acid oils, and their heightened metabolism requires higher amounts of the energy foods—starches. This is the normal pattern of childhood.

If a child observes her parents eating nourishing foods and she is frequently offered them but not forced to eat them, she will eventually incorporate these foods into her diet. This change is gradual and usually occurs in the middle to late teens. I urge you not to force a child to eat like you too early. This results in a "power struggle," which may delay the child's normal dietary progression.

If children do not observe their parents consuming nutritious foods and refusing unwholesome ones, a pattern of malnourishment is sure to follow. A child will continue the normal dietary pattern of childhood well into adulthood, consuming high amounts of fat and starch, leading to the imbalance of essential nutrients, which, in turn, leads to the development of many health syndromes. Just as children must be taught how to work, they must be taught how to eat in this modern world of junk- and fast-food options.

The next time you go to your grocery store, observe the package design of the processed and junk foods. I think you will find they are designed for children. This industry knows a customer early in childhood is a customer for life. The tobacco industry knows this advertising principle also and uses it to our country's great detriment.

Every parent knows the relentless energy of a child. Over time it is tempting to give in to their persistent requests for sweets and sodas. I urge you to not give in but to compromise. Try to make routine snacks nutritious and fun for children. Have a birthday cake on their special day, but don't celebrate fifty-two birthdays per year.

I have found that children readily accept explanations and are eager to learn about what is good for them. Nature gives us all a sense of survival, and children are no exception. I can think of no greater gift to your child than the skills needed to lead an independent, healthy life.

If your childhood has passed and you know changes are needed, do not give up hope. It has been my observation that even experienced senior citizens have the ability to change and benefit from that change. The most important factor for us to change, is the desire to do so.

THE GREATEST GIFT A PARENT CAN GIVE A CHILD IS THE ABILITY TO LIVE AN INDEPENDENT, HEALTHY LIFE.

One of the most gratifying aspects of being a family doctor is watching children grow into hearty productive adulthood. I have listed some common-sense pointers for you to consider in your foundation for prevention.

Rx _____

A Foundation for Prevention for Children

1. Start your baby's life with nutritious and immune-supportive breast milk for the first six months of life or longer whenever possible.

2. Newborns and infants cry for specific reasons. Pain, hunger, thirst, a dirty or wet diaper, and the need for love and attention are all normal causes of crying. If your baby continues to cry after addressing these basic needs, there is a problem that

needs addressing. If your investigation yields no apparent cause, seek the help of your health care professional. Babies under two years of age are not yet capable of manipulating you into action. In other words, babies under two years of age do not cry because they are spoiled. After two, this all begins to change.

3. Allow your child to have only one immunization at a time. This may be a combination vaccine like DPT. To give an infant two or three injections at a time, containing six to eight immunizations, is cruel and capable of causing violent reactions in a child. Spacing the immunizations two weeks apart takes more time and money but is in the best interest of your child's health.

4. Provide a basic multiple-vitamin supplement for your child as soon as possible. Dietary patterns are established early in life. The daily ritual of taking a vitamin for their health establishes a pattern for life.

5. At six months of age introduce one new food at a time and wait at least one week before starting another, watching for signs of food allergies. Start with a simple low-allergy food like rice cereal.

6. Include your children as early as possible in your pursuit of spiritual fitness. Teach them your family's religious heritage, for they are eager to learn of our higher power.

7. Cow's milk is not necessary for proper growth and development and is the most common cause of food allergies.

8. Obtain a quality water filter to improve the flavor of your water and encourage its consumption.

9. Dehydration is infants' and toddlers' worst enemy. Dehydration alone can cause a significant rise in temperature. A well-hydrated child has a far greater chance of healing quickly.

10. An ill, dehydrated baby has a dry mouth, makes few tears, and infrequently wets his/her diaper. Start to hydrate with sips of hydrating solutions or water. Advance slowly. A child can go much longer without food than water. Be sure the child can hold water before attempting a feeding.

11. During a febrile illness do not attempt to drive the fever below 100 degrees. To do so may delay healing and require too much medication.

12. Make a practice of asking your family doctor or pediatrician if an antibiotic is really needed for your child's illness. More often than not febrile illnesses do not require antibiotics. If the child fails to progress on schedule, notify your doctor so that any changes may be instituted. During and after antibiotic therapy, provide yogurt with extra acidophilus added. Strictly avoid sugar during antibiotic use to avoid the overgrowth of candida.

13. Any fever higher than 103 degrees should be evaluated by a health care professional.

14. A health care professional should evaluate any fever greater than 101 degrees that lasts for more than three days.

15. If your child becomes profoundly ill in a short period of time (within minutes), seek immediate medical attention.

16. Your toddler will give you clues when it is time to start toilet training. They do not like to be messy any more than you like changing diapers. Girls tend to show the desire to be free of diapers before boys. Starting the toilet training process too early to SATISFY THE PARENTS will prolong the training

period and create stress for both child and parents. A toddler will provide you with behavioral clues when it is time to start toilet training. Provide fun rewards for dry training pants and a toddler's requests to be taken to the restroom. Never punish a toddler for having a toilet training accident.

17. An injured child who does not cry requires immediate careful attention. Children who cry vigorously after a fall are usually not seriously injured, and their primary need is to be consoled.

18. Every child has his or her own unique tempo of growth, development, and maturation. Growth spurts can come at varied times, even among children of the same parents.

19. It is normal for a child to be sleepy and nauseated after a bump on the head. He may be allowed to sleep, but he should be responsive if you arouse him. Confusion, unequal pupils, and protracted vomiting are danger signs that warrant evaluation by a health care professional.

20. Help your children with their homework, and be involved in activities that support the school. You may be surprised how much algebra you remember.

Home tutoring stresses the importance of education and tells your children of your concern for their future.

21. Encourage outside play.

22. Limit computer games and encourage interactive physical games.

23. Limit television, and do not allow television in the child's room.

24. If you purchase junk food and bring it into the home, children will eat it. Soda and sweet fruit drinks are a leading cause of childhood obesity. Do not make them a part of your child's daily diet.

25. Support your child's athletic ambitions with the understanding that not all children are athletic, just as not all adults are athletic. After a good try at sports, a frustrated child should not be forced to continue.

26. Try to have at least one meal a day together as a family.

27. Have a bowl of nuts and seeds along with fresh fruit available for the kids when they come home from school.

28. Teach your children how to work by making them responsible for their own laundry and the upkeep of their rooms and assorted tasks around the home as soon as possible. You can do too much for a child. It is usually easier to do these things yourself, but the child will pay a price for your work later in life.

29. Most adolescents go through some difficult times. Be patient.

30. In many school districts the cafeterias now serve meals of fast-food quality. Take the time to prepare a sack lunch for your children to eat at school. As kids reach junior high and high school, make the preparation of their sack lunches their responsibility, if this is practical. This way adolescents will recognize and be responsible for their own dietary needs.

31. If you have more than one child, spend some "quality time" with each child individually. This confirms a child's uniqueness and helps develop a strong parent/child bond for the rest of your lives.

32. Try to console your children or reward them for good behavior with something other than junk food. Junk-food rewards can set up a pattern of inappropriate eating for life.

33. Be a good example to your children in selecting and eating a healthful diet, while refusing unhealthful foods.

Richard L. Becker, .D.O.

Rx

A FOUNDATION FOR PREVENTION FOR ADULTS

1. If you are facing health challenges, start with the HEALING DIET and progress via the TRANSITIONAL DIET to the DIET FOR THE REST OF YOUR LIFE.

2. If you are in good health, start with the DIET FOR THE REST OF YOUR LIFE.

3. You may adapt the DIET FOR THE REST OF YOUR LIFE to your personal needs and taste. Be a vegetarian if you wish, but if that is the diet you prefer it is imperative that you strictly avoid refined grains and sugars in your daily routine. Excessive consumption of refined sugars and starches is the most common dietary mistake vegetarians make. Vegetarians should also supplement vitamin B 12 as deficiencies of this vitamin

is relatively common in those who consume only plant based foods. Whether you choose to be vegetarian or not, include soy in its varied forms in your diet as the soy bean is a source of complete protein and understand what other vegetarian foods may be combined for a source of complete protein. The following food groups when eaten together make a source of complete protein: grains with nuts and seeds, grains with legumes, grains with milk products, nuts and seeds with legumes, nuts and seeds with milk.

4. Eat "in season" as much as possible. When apples come to harvest in the fall, consume them daily, but eat them sparingly during other seasons. Use this example for all the varied fruits, vegetables, and grains, including breads. Cyclic consumption of fruits, vegetables, and grains is the historical use of these foods. You do not need extended time off from any food; just try to find a cycle that fits your needs. This practice helps assure a wide variety of foods is consumed at their peak state for nutrition—fresh from the garden. Meats, fish, legumes, dairy, nuts, and seeds do not need to be consumed in a cycle and can be eaten daily.

5. Do not make refined white flour of any grain part of your daily routine.

6. Avoid prepackaged, refined, and processed foods.

7. Do not include cured and salted meats in your daily routine.

8. Consume a variety of raw leafy and different-colored vegetables daily.

9. Juice with tart, low-sugar fruits and vegetables at least two times a week.

10. Avoid fast-food restaurants completely. If this simple statement isn't sufficiently convincing, go into any of the nationwide fast-food chain establishments and ask to see the exact ingredients of each food offered. The list of ingredients in a simple hamburger bun is staggering and requires an advanced degree in chemistry to understand. Cafeterias are a better fast-food option.

11. Never skip breakfast. This pattern is the most consistent feature of those who are battling obesity. Eat breakfast within thirty minutes of rising in the morning. Breakfast should be a balanced meal built around protein-rich foods.

12. Three meals and a snack are appropriate for most people. You may need four meals and a snack. Two

meals a day is rarely a wholesome option as the practice leads to overeating during the last meal.

13. Drink 1/2 oz of chlorine-free water per pound of body weight a day. Any tea or coffee is extra.

14. Limit coffee to no more than two cups a day, and consider drinking tea in its place.

15. Do not drink carbonated beverages or sweet fruit flavored drinks as a daily routine.

16. Exercise for at least twenty minutes four times a week. Walking, swimming, and biking are the least damaging to your joints. Many people prefer exercise that includes a ball. If this helps you get the exercise you need, play tennis, golf, or basketball. Have options available for bad-weather days. An established pattern of exercise should not be brought to a halt by one cold front. Develop hobbies that include exercise such as gardening.

17. Wear sunglasses while driving and outdoors to protect your eyes from cataract-causing sunlight.

18. Expose your skin to sunlight as healthy levels of vitamin D help protect us from cancer, heart disease and osteoporosis. However, never allow your skin to

become sunburned. Wear sunscreen and protective clothing and a hat during prolonged outdoor activity.

19. Limit alcohol intake to two drinks or less daily, and never use any form of tobacco.

20. Never eat margarine, and limit cow's milk intake, but consume frequent servings of butter, cottage cheese, buttermilk, cream cheese, yogurt, and sour cream.

21. Recognize early in life that humans are spiritual beings. Exercise your "spiritual muscles" just as you exercise your body's muscles.

22. The growth and development of life continues, cradle to grave. Accept the changing roles that maturity brings. As we age, families and communities look to senior citizens for wisdom and gentle guidance. This is a tremendous opportunity to have a positive impact on young people's lives, while fulfilling personal needs for continued growth.

23. Know what the essential nutritional elements of life are and supplement them daily in your diet. Protein, essential fatty acids, the antioxidant vitamins A, C, and E, the B vitamins, minerals, and trace minerals are all essential. A high potency multiple vitamin, mineral and

amino acid powder will provide all the known essential dietary elements with the exception of the fatty acids. A variety of multiple vitamin powders are commercially available today that include extracts of fruits and vegetables known to be of benefit to your health.

24. If you have a health condition become aware of which conditionally essential nutrients may help improve your health status. Conditionally essential nutrients are normally made by our bodies but with age, injury or during times of illness their production may become compromised. For example, coenzyme Q10, L-carnitine and D-ribose are all conditionally essential nutrients and heart disease patients often benefit from their supplementation. This area of nutritional research is quickly expanding and holds great promise for our health and welfare.

25. Make learning about health a priority in life. Dedicate one hour a week to reading, watching, or listening to health issues.

26. Understand that we are all responsible for our actions. If your doctor offers you a prescription medication, ask if there is an effective nonmedication alternative. If there is no viable alternative, be familiar with the potential side effects the medication may cause.

27. The use of alternative and holistic health practices does not exclude the use of medications and surgery. The best approach is to integrate all that science validates. Use diet, exercise, supplements and spiritual fulfillment to prevent disease. If disease strikes, use modern medicine to manage the crisis while integrating holistic measures as soon as possible to help you heal.

28. Vitamins, minerals, various supplements, and herbs, though in general well-tolerated, may have side effects. A skilled health care provider should supervise large dosages of any supplement.

29. Choose a source of essential fatty acids such as fish oil, oil of primrose, flaxseed oil, perilla, or borage seed oil and take 2–4 grams daily. By rotating through the list of essential fatty acid supplements, you will find the one that suits you best. You may also obtain a product that combines several sources of essential fatty acids. They are all helpful and none of them is a mistake. Replace a portion of the calories received from starchy foods in the diet with vegetable oils, such as olive and sunflower seed oil.

30. Add a fiber supplement to your high-fiber diet. Glucomannan and psyllium are excellent choices, but oat bran and prunes are also good. Even a synthetic fiber such as calcium polycarbophil or methylcellulose

may be helpful if you find the natural sources cause bloating or gas.

31. Seek out a nutritionally minded family physician as your primary health care giver. Do not try to manage specialty doctors by yourself.

32. Use the following list of supplements as a foundation for prevention:

a. High potency multiple vitamin, mineral and amino acid powder: 1 tbs daily.

b. Noni juice: 1–4 oz daily.

c. Coenzyme Q10: 10–30 mg daily.

d. Oligomeric proanthocyanidins (OPC) with at least 95% active component purity: 100 mg daily.

e. Fish or flaxseed oil: 2 grams daily.

f. Glucosamine sulfate: 300 mg 2 tablets daily.

g. Chondroitin sulfate: 200 mg 2 tablets daily.

h. Methylsulfonylmethane (MSM): 300 mg 2 tablets daily.

i. Gingko biloba: 240 mg daily (do not take with warfarin or any other blood thinning agent).

j. Cereal grass or green food extract (barley, wheat, oat, spirulina, etc.): 2 grams daily.

k. Sea kelp: 1 gram daily or an alternate source of trace minerals.

l. Maintain beneficial intestinal bacteria by eating raw fruits and vegetables daily, sauerkraut, fermented diary products, such as yogurt, and by taking probiotic supplements routinely.

m. Beta glucan: 3 mg, 1 capsule daily at bedtime for immune support.

n. Address your family's medical history and your increased risk of developing familial diseases by selecting appropriate supplements listed in the section concerning the treatment of those conditions.

Richard L. Becker, .D.O.

27

SENIOR HEALTH

America is aging and contrary to belief the process is not a disease. There are more American senior citizens alive today than ever before. In fact of all the people who have lived to be 65 years of age over one-half of them are alive today. Opportunities for seniors exist as never before –extended life, political recognition and power, travel, economic stability and time with family and friends. Yet so many still are burdened with degenerative health conditions that greatly compromise their continued growth and fulfillment during these golden years. The majority of us have worked hard our entire adult life with the hope of some day retiring in health and comfort. The bulk of America's senior's financial resources is now being dedicated to ever increasing doctor and pharmacy bills as sixty percent of the total health care spending today is by seniors.

The physiologic effects of aging are a normal part of life however the degenerative aspects of aging can be greatly accelerated if healthy lifestyle practices are not in place. Years of poor dietary and exercise habits begin to take their toll. Minor annoyances of middle age evolve into disease processes that cause pain and greatly compromise quality of life. Many turn to medications falsely believing it is their only hope in regaining their youthful vitality. Seven of every ten pills made in America are taken by senior citizens. Is successful aging just about taking medications? Weekly visits to the internist and pharmacist is not what we have diligently worked and saved for.

"Follow the whole instruction the Lord your God has commanded you, so that you may live, prosper and have a long life in the land you will possess."
                                                    Deuteronomy 5:33

It is a common notion with advancing age come inevitable disability. This attitude is to often held by doctors. Many of you after expressing a complaint to your physician have heard, "Well Mrs. Jones you are 82 years old and with age comes many challenges. Let's try a new medication and see if it helps". Rarely, does the doctor inquire into dietary and lifestyle practices nor does he recommend vitamins or supplements even though volumes of scientific writings validate their use in seniors. The ancient practice of physicians sharing holistic wisdom with their aged patients has now been replaced with one pill prescription after another –at a time in life when seniors need knowledge the most.

The following list of recommendations and guidelines have helped many seniors regain their youthful vitality. In fact many who follow this plan report they feel better at 70 than they did at 30 years of age. I urge you, America's seniors, to embrace the years ahead of you. Face them with the same dignity, style and grace that allowed you to mature into the complete wise person you are today.

> *"For by wisdom your days will be many, and years will be added to your life."*
>
> Proverbs 9:11

Rx _____

RECOMMENDATIONS AND GUIDELINES
FOR AGING GRAGEFULLY

1. ***Seniors, we must be aware that our bodies are different now. The aging process causes our bodies to react to disease differently.*** With age, organs most affected by past health problems often display symptoms even if the current health condition is not

involving that symptom. For example: The elderly patient who has hyperthyroidism may not have an enlarged thyroid gland or a tremor but rather they will show confusion, depression, fainting and weakness. The elderly patient with pneumonia may not have a cough with fever but rather confusion, fainting and urinary incontinence. If you feel the least bit confused, dizzy, and depressed or if you have developed any form of incontinence or have fainting spells please have a thorough checkup as these symptoms are common signs of an underlying health problem in seniors. This phenomenon often leads patients and doctors down a diagnostic pathway investigating the organ systems displaying these general symptoms when the real culprit resides in a completely different area.

2. *As we age our organ systems do not have the depth of reserve they once did. This leads to the development of disease symptom very early in the course of disease.* For example: In the elderly, heart failure may be precipitated by a very mild case of hyperthyroidism. The hyperthyroidism may be so mild, if a young person should have the same degree of hyperthyroidism, they would not have any cardiac symptoms. With an elderly person they may be confined to bed with shortness of breath, chest pain

and fluid retention. If a senior man with an enlarged prostate takes an over the counter cold medication it may cause a spike of blood pressure and difficulty in urination. Although this phenomenon creates dramatic symptoms when disease strikes it also draws attention to the disease. If proper treatment is started or medication adjustments are made a simple change often leads to dramatic improvement in overall health and vitality for the senior. Unfortunately seniors and doctors frequently accept these accentuated symptoms as a part of the aging process. When in reality it is an early warning of disease that if addressed early on may help avoid tragedy.

3. *If a senior has an incurable health condition even a minor problem in another organ system can greatly aggravate the incurable condition.* For example; a person with early Alzheimer's disease who develops a bladder infection will show a dramatic increase in combativeness, confusion and disorientation; symptoms common in end stage Alzheimer's disease. Or the senior with advance spinal stenosis and chronic pain who becomes acutely constipated will often develop a spike in their pain syndrome. Since these patient's primary condition is incurable, patient and doctor alike may think nothing can be done to improve the patient's condition; when in fact

proper treatment for the co-existing, aggravating malady usually leads to dramatic improvement in the "incurable" disease.

4. Loss of appetite, pain, confusion, anemia, depression, insomnia, fatigue, irregularity, incontinence and feeling poorly in general are not a part of the normal aging process. It should not be accepted but rather investigated and the underlying cause corrected whenever possible.

5. *Because senior's depth of strength is compromised the prevention of disease continues to play a paramount role in promoting health.* For example; since cardiovascular disease is the leading cause of death in seniors, controlling hypertension, body weight and staying fit continues to play a vital role in promoting both quality and quantity of life. Since osteoporosis and hip fracture is a leading cause of long term hospitalization and death for seniors, supplementing the diet with calcium and minerals along with engaging in stability strengthening exercises also continues to play a vital role in preventing falls and broken bones.

6. The most common causes of senior disability include arthritis, falls and injury, cardiovascular disease, cancer, diabetes and visual impairment. If you

have gained weight or have virtually any ongoing health condition that compromises your vitality, for best results, refer to the chapters or suggested readings that discuss these conditions and follow the recommendations listed. If you are doing well and your weight is ideal follow THE DIET FOR THE REST OF YOUR LIFE.

7. With advancing age chewing whole protein rich foods may become difficult. Many seniors replace meats and other protein rich foods with sugary and fatty soft foods. Be careful as this may aggravate or cause diabetes. Eggs, chopped meats, stews and soups, protein powder supplements and nut butters offer easy to chew protein rich foods. Juicing and puréeing fruits and vegetables allow easy consumption of healthy plant based foods. Dentures should fit well and not cause any oral sores as loose or irritating dentures may compromise feedings.

8. Chronic dehydration greatly accelerates the aging process. Unless your doctor has specifically instructed you to restrict water consumption, drink more water. Drink 1/2 ounce of chlorine free water per pound of body weight.

9. The average American senior consumes 3-5 times the recommended salt intake. This practice can aggravate hypertension and heart failure along with increasing your medication dependency. Unprocessed whole foods are naturally low in sodium and allowed. Avoid daily consumption of prepackaged salted snacks and salted or cured meats. Strive for an average of no more than 3,000 mg of salt intake daily.

10. Exercise is a vital part of your plan for continued wellness. Multiple medical studies have shown seniors who make exercise a part of their daily life have less depression, pain, heart disease, diabetes and overall disability. Further, seniors who exercise, consistently report they are more content with their lives, while feeling better able to face the challenges of aging. In

THE DAY YOU RESIGN YOURSELF TO PASS AWAY RETIREMENT IN A ROCKING CHAIR IS THE BEGINNING OF THE FINAL CHAPTER OF YOUR LIFE.

fact seniors who exercise have twice the life expectancy compared to seniors who do not exercise. Safe exercise options include: walking, stationary cycling, swimming and resistance weight training. Also include stability and trunk strengthening exercises to help avoid falls. Your physician can refer you to a physical therapist who will help develop a plan to meet your specific needs.

11. As we age our ability to absorb essential nutrients becomes compromised which in turn greatly accelerates the degenerative processes of aging. Deficiencies of the B vitamins, vitamins A and D, calcium and iron are the most common nutrient deficiencies in seniors and these nutrients should be supplemented daily. Do not take high doses of iron unless specifically instructed to by your physician. The amount of iron in a multiple vitamin (10 mg or less) is allowed and encouraged.

12. Free radical damage plays a major role in premature aging. Eating fresh fruits and vegetables daily along with supplementing the antioxidant vitamins and minerals will help prevent needless free radical damage. A high potency multiple vitamin, mineral and amino acid powder: 1 tbs daily will supply the essential nutrients discussed in numbers 11 and 12.

13. If you have or are at high risk for osteoporosis refer to Chapter 24—OSTEOPOROSIS and follow the instructions listed. For maximum absorbable mineral intake add to your high potency multiple vitamin, mineral and amino acid powder, microcrystalline hydroxyapatite (bone meal): 6 capsules daily for a total of 2000 mg calcium daily.

14. Fish or flaxseed oil with borage seed oil: 2 grams of each daily.

15. Coenzyme Q10/L-carnitine: 30 mg/250 mg daily for cardiac energy.

16. Alpha lipoic acid: 300 mg daily for efficient blood glucose metabolism.

17. Grape seed-extracted oliogomeric proanthocyanidins (OPC) with at least 95% active component purity: 200 mg daily for vascular integrity.

18. Lutein: 3 mg daily for eye health

19. Zeaxanthine: .3 mg daily for eye health

20. Glucomannan fiber: 575 mg 4-6 capsules daily for regularity.

21. Probiotics with fructo-oligosaccharides: 1 tablet daily for intestinal health.

22. Melatonin: 3 mg 1-6 tablets at bedtime for sleep, as needed.

23. Be sure the home is free of clutter and obstructions and all walk ways are well lighted. Falls are the sixth leading cause of death in seniors and they are a contributing factor in forty percent of nursing home admissions. One out of four falls result in serious injury and five percent result in a bone fracture. Exercise, stability strengthening, canes and ambulatory assistance devices, vitamin D, vitamin B 12 and folate have all been shown to help reduce the occurrence of falls in seniors and calcium supplements help to preserve bone strength.

24. Seniors are three times more likely to suffer side effects from medications. All medications have side effects including over the counter drugs. The following list of medications are the medications most likely to cause side effects in seniors. Sleeping pills and sedatives of any type (Valium, Ativan, Lunesta etc.), narcotic pain medication, non-narcotic pain medication such as the non-steroidal anti-inflammatory agents (aspirin, ibuprofen, naproxen, Celebrex etc.), antibiotics, digoxin, diuretics, beta blockers (propranolol, Tenormin, Toprol-XL, Blocadren, Brevibloc), cimetidine (Tagamet), steroids (prednisone, cortisone, dexamethasone etc.) antidepressants, glaucoma medications and anticoagulants such as warfarin. Many seniors do

take these medications without difficulty. Please be aware of their potential risk and know your ability to tolerate them may change.

25. A compartmentalized daily medication dispenser will help assure you that you are taking your medications as prescribed. Simply put your medications in their daily compartment, take them as prescribed and at the end of the day check to be sure the compartment is empty.

26. Many seniors look forward to traveling during retirement. Consider these tips while making your travel plans:

    a. If you want to get away, fall is the perfect time to do so. You won't have to deal with big crowds and travel is less expensive.

    b. If leaving the country, be sure your passport is up to date.

    c. Inform a friend or family member of your travel itinerary.

    d. Many countries around the world have diseases you are not familiar with. Consult your physician for medical clearance and proper immunization.

e. Use a suitcase with wheels and a pulling handle so that it is easy to move it about. Many travelers have strained their spine by lifting and carrying heavy luggage.

f. Be sure you have enough medication and supplements to last the entire trip plus a few extra days in case you encounter any travel delays. Carry your medications in their original prescription bottle with you on the plane so you always have your medications even if your luggage is lost.

g. Medication dosage times during travel can be confusing. If your medications are time sensitive and the trip is 2 days or shorter take your medications based on the time at home. If the trip is longer than 2 days adapt your dosage time to the local time.

h. If you require a wheelchair or an ambulatory assistance device notify the airport and your hotel so they may provide any special services you may require. Wear a medical condition bracelet or pendant to inform others of your condition in case you are unable to provide a medical history.

i. Protect yourself from infections by washing your hands or use an alcohol-based "hand sanitizer" after spending time on a plane, train or bus.

j. Be careful of what you eat and drink. Traveler's diarrhea can ruin a much anticipated trip. Drink bottled water and avoid raw foods in areas of poor sanitation.

k. Become aware of your destination's medical facilities and whether they accept your health insurance.

l. Air travel causes dehydration and promotes poor circulation. Drink plenty of water and get up out your chair and move as frequently as possible. Wearing support stockings and engaging in isotonic exercises by flexing the leg and calf muscles while seated also helps to prevent blood pooling.

m. In general flying west induces less jet lag than flying east. Take this into account by scheduling rest days when making travel plans. Melatonin: 3-24 mg prior to bed after travel reduces jet lag.

27. As we age our body's reflex time increases creating hazards while driving automobiles. The AARP Safe Driving Program, formerly known as 55ALIVE, teaches seniors driving techniques to compensate for these delayed reaction times. These skills will help assure your safety and prolong your independence. Call 1-888-227-7669 for a course near you.

28. Health screenings continue to play a vital role in disease prevention. The following list summarizes the U.S Preventive Services Task Force recommended disease screening tests for healthy adults:

    a. Screening mammography with or without clinical breast examination every 1-2 years for women aged 40 and older.

    b. Screening Pap smears every 1-3 years for women who have a cervix and are sexually active. Women over 65 do not need Pap smears if they have had past Pap smears that did not show abnormalities and they are not at high risk for cervical cancer.

    c. Screening for colorectal cancer may be conducted annually by home fecal occult blood testing. Colorectal cancer screening may also be conducted with flexible sigmoidoscopy or double-contrast barium enema every 5 years or by colonoscopy every 10 years.

29. Although not universally agreed upon many doctors recommend the following health screening tests or immunizations for seniors:

    a. Prostate specific antigen testing along with digital prostate exam every 2-3 years.

b. Skin cancer screening exams for those at high risk (prior skin cancer, fair skinned, multiple moles, a history of multiple sun burns, or a family history of skin cancer) every 1-3 years.

c. Eye exams for early detection of macular degeneration, cataract formation and glaucoma every 1-2 years.

d. Complete blood count, serum chemistry with cholesterol and lipid profile, thyroid function, serum vitamin B12 and folate levels and urine analysis every 1-2 years.

e. Yearly influenza immunization for those with diabetes, heart or lung disease or those who live in a nursing home facility.

f. Pneumonia immunization for those with diabetes, heart or lung disease or those who live in a nursing home facility.

30. When you visit the doctor take all your medications and dietary supplements with you so the doctor is fully aware of what you are taking. Remember; seniors are very sensitive to medications. Just because you have tolerated a

medication in the past does not mean it is not the cause of your troubles today.

31. In preparation for a doctor visit write down how you feel and any questions you may have and take the list with you to the doctor's office. Take notes during the office visit if appropriate and ask for written instructions from the doctor. If this becomes too difficult bring a family member or friend with you to help you keep track of the details.

32. Human growth and development continues from cradle to grave. Stay involved by maintaining social interaction with family and friends, church attendance, reading and spiritual study for as long as possible. Your community could benefit from your experience in life. Volunteering is a great way to share your knowledge while staying involved. I can not over-state the vital importance of these activities. Contact Points of Light Foundation at 1-800-750-7653 for volunteer opportunities in your town.

33. By completing an advanced health care directive and appointing a durable power of attorney for health care you will be assured that the care provided you follows your wishes even if you are unable to express them.

34. Many retirement and assisted living centers are in operation today. These centers are designed to meet the needs of active, independent seniors. By relieving the burden of home maintenance and the preparation of meals and promoting social interaction, these centers are capable of extending a senior's quality of life. If this is a viable option for you visit several centers before the need arises so that you can make a wise choice.

35. A small minority of seniors resides in a nursing home; however, making plans for this possibility, or an alternative, and including these plans in your advanced health care directive will assure your wishes are followed.

Richard L. Becker, .D.O.

Neil M. Resnick, M.D., Harrison's Principles of Internal Medicine 14th Edition, Geriatric Medicine

Ferdinando L. Mirarchi, D.O., What's the Patient's Code Status? P.A.E.R.

RESOURCES

It has always been a concern that my patients are not getting the absolute best quality supplements available. Most of the multiple vitamin and mineral preparations on the market are poorly formulated and incapable of providing maximum safe benefit. Our bodies require nutrients that are complimented by other nutrients at specific ratios for proper utilization. For example, calcium requires the presence of magnesium and other trace minerals to be efficiently absorbed from the intestinal tract and deposited in bone tissue. Taking just calcium alone may result in constipation and nausea. Thereby limiting its effectiveness and the likelihood of continued supplementation of a mineral we all know is needed on a daily basis. Thus the challenge of vitamin and mineral therapy is to develop formulations that accurately reflect nature's intended nutrients, in balance, and in an organic absorbable form.

The scientific evidence points to the chelation of essential nutrients as the very best method of vitamin and mineral formulation for your daily dose of multiple vitamins and minerals. Nature attaches nutrients to protein amino acids and organic Kreb cycle molecules by means of normal plant physiology. By extracting and concentrating these molecules and including them in our vitamins and mineral regimen we achieve maximum safe nutrient dosage that is slowly released throughout the day affording low levels of nausea and prohibitive side effects while achieving maximum nutrition.

The high potency multiple vitamin, mineral and amino acid blends, DR. BECKER'S BIONUTRIENTS are the result of many years of research and clinical experience. Family doctors are very practical people; our therapies must work and they must be as free from side effects as possible. This has been the guiding principle in the development of these maximum potency blends. Over the years, hundreds of my patients have benefited from these remarkable formulas. I urge you to consider DR. BECKER'S BIONUTRIENTS when purchasing your next multiple vitamin. Available in four blends, Organic Green, Berry, Active Adult and Low Allergy Rice DR. BECKER'S BIONUTRIENTS has a formula to meet your nutritional needs.

For the very best results always take DR. BECKER'S BIONUTRIENTS after a meal. Mix up to one heaping tablespoon in a small glass of water or juice. Immediately following the dosage, drink a large glass of water, and then drink another glass of water one hour later. Never take any multiple vitamins on an empty stomach. Far too many skip breakfast and take their supplements on an empty stomach. Extracted vitamins and minerals are concentrated nutrients. Nature always provides fiber and buffering agents in foods and you should do the same with your vitamin and mineral blends by taking them after a meal.

Most vitamin and mineral deficiency states require several weeks of treatment to fully correct. Give your supplement program a little time before passing judgment. In our fast paced world obtaining maximum nutrition from just food is a difficult goal to achieve. Vitamin and mineral supplementation is a good idea for even the healthy.

DR. BECKER'S BIONUTRIENTS are available direct from BIO INNOVATIONS, P.O. BOX 2485, Rockwall, Texas 75087, and 888.442.5150 or at www.bioinnovations.net.

Cindy, my wife, and I developed ALOHA NONI JUICE to fill a need for fresh, sugar free Noni juice, at a price people could afford. Morinda citrifolia (Noni) is most effective when taken fresh, as it has been used for thousands of years. Mixing fresh Noni juice with a fruit juice of your choice will help cover it's strong pungent taste. I suggest mixing Noni with red grape juice or a tropical fruit juice like mango or papaya. ALOHA NONI JUICE is available direct from BIO INNOVATIONS, P.O. BOX 2485, Rockwall, Texas 75087, and 888.442.5150 or at www.alohanoni.com.

NONI NATURALS is an elegant line of skin care products that feature Polynesian Noni, beta glucan, and many therapeutic herbal ingredients. One of Noni's most remarkable uses is it's application to skin. NONI NATURALS offers a complete system of skin care and is available direct from BIO INNOVATIONS, P.O. BOX 2485, Rockwall, Texas 75087, and 888.442.5150 or at www.bioinnovations.net.

IMMUNE POWER liquid supplement: to order call 888-741-LIFE

DR. BECKER'S WEIGHT LOSS SOLUTION MEAL REPLACEMENT PROGRAM is available direct from BIO INNOVATIONS, P.O. BOX 2485, Rockwall, Texas 75087, and 888.442.5150 or at www.bioinnovations.net.

The supplements listed in this book are generally available at fine health food stores. Most of them are available direct from BIO INNOVATIONS, P.O. BOX 2485, Rockwall, Texas 75087, and 888.442.5150 or at www.alohanoni.com.

Suggested Reading List

1. Patrick Quillin, Ph.D., R.D., C.N.S. with Noreen Quillin, *Beating Cancer with Nutrition*, Nutrition Times Press, Inc.

2. Michael Murray, N.D. and Joseph Pizzorno, N.D., *Encyclopedia of Natural Medicine*, Revised 2nd Edition. Prima Health.

3. Phyllis A. Balch, C.N.C. and James F. Balch, M.D., *Prescription for Nutritional Healing*, 3rd Edition. Avery.

4. Sheldon Saul Hendler, Ph.D., M.D. and David Rorvik, M.S., Chief Editors, *Physicians' Desk Reference for Nutritional Supplements*, Medical Economics.

5. Richard N. Firshein, D.O., *The Nutraceutical Revolution*, Riverhead Books.

6. Thomas Fleming, R.Ph. Chief Editor, *Physicians' Desk Reference for Herbal Medicines*, Medical Economics Company.

7. Jacob Teitelbaum, M.D., *From Fatigued to Fantastic*, Avery.

8. Jacob Teitelbaum, M.D., *Pain Free 1-2-3!*, Deva Press.

9. Stephen T. Sinatra, M.D., F.A.C.C., *The Sinatra Solution, Metabolic Cardiology*, Basic Health Publications.

10. Nancy Appleton, Ph.D., *Lick the Sugar Habit*, Avery.

11. Boris Draznin, M.D., Ph.D., *The Draznin Plan, The Thinking Person's Guide to Diabetes*, Oxford University Press.

12. Steven Bratman, M.D., with David Kroll, Ph.D., *Natural Health Bible*, Prima Health.

13. Ferdinando L. Mirarchi, D.O., *What's the Patient's Code Status?* P.A.E.R.

END NOTES

1. Elie Metchnikoff, Ph.D., *The Prolongation of Life*, G. P. Putnam's Sons, 1908, p. 161.

2. <u>A. V. Valyshev, L. S.Zykova, M. E. Konnova</u>. [The screening diagnosis of intestinal dysbiosis] Zh Mikrobiol Epidemiol Immunobiol. Suppl 1, Aug-Sep 1994:71–74. Russian. PMID: 7856356 [PubMed—indexed for MEDLINE].

3. <u>A. V. Valyshev, F. G. Gil'mutdinova, A. A. Tret'iakov, S. V. Fomicheva, O. V. Bukharin</u>. [The role of persisting opportunistic intestinal microflora in dysbiosis in the occurrence of hepatobiliary system diseases] Zh Mikrobiol Epidemiol Immunobiol. 4 (Jul–Aug 1997):87–88. Russian. PMID: 9341011 [PubMed—indexed for MEDLINE].

4. A. V. Valyshev, F. G. Gil'mutdinova, S. V. Fomicheva.
[The persistence factors of the enterobacteria in the fecal flora in intestinal dysbiosis] Zh Mikrobiol Epidemiol Immunobiol. 3 (May–Jun 1996):96–98. Russian. PMID: 8771745 [PubMed—indexed for MEDLINE].

5. E. M. Gorskaia, L. G. Zaitseva, V. M. Bondarenko, E. I. Vasil'eva, O. I. U. Kornienko, L. N. Mazankova.
[The Amben regulation of the intestinal microflora and macrophage functional activity in an experiment] Zh Mikrobiol Epidemiol Immunobiol. 1 (Jan–Feb 1995):87–90. Russian. PMID: 7778385 [PubMed—indexed for MEDLINE].

6. S. K. Kanareykina, A. A. Misautova, A. R. Zlatkina, E. N. Levina.
Proteus dysbioses in patients with ulcerative colitis. Nahrung. 1987;31(5-6)(1987):557–561. PMID: 3657933 [PubMed—indexed for MEDLINE].

7. E. A. Lykova, V. M. Bondarenko, A. A. Vorob'ev, E. V. Sudzhan, V. I. Minaev, V. E. Malikov.
[Bacterial endotoxinemia in children with intestinal dysbacteriosis] Zh Mikrobiol Epidemiol Immunobiol. 3 (May–Jun 1999):67–70. Russian. PMID: 10851996 [PubMed—indexed for MEDLINE].

8. S. S. Gizatulina, M. O. Birger, M. I. Nikovskaia, I.
   U. N. Mastiukova, L. A. Potashova.
   [Intestinal microflora in young children with
   rotavirus infection] Zh Mikrobiol Epidemiol
   Immunobiol. 3 (Mar 1992):29–30. Russian. PMID:
   1509842 [PubMed—indexed for MEDLINE].

9. N. M. Gracheva, A. F. Gavrilov, A. I. Solov'eva, V.
   V. Smirnov, I. B. Sorokulova, S. R. Reznik, N. V.
   Chudnovskaia.
   [The efficacy of the new bacterial preparation
   biosporin in treating acute intestinal infections] Zh
   Mikrobiol Epidemiol Immunobiol. 1(Jan–Feb 1996):
   75–77. Russian. PMID: 8820685 [PubMed—indexed
   for MEDLINE].

10. Z. E. Lineva.
    [Clinical and bacteriological features of intestinal
    dysbacteriosis in patients with pulmonary
    tuberculosis] Probl Tuberk. 2(1997):27–28. Russian.
    PMID: 9235578 [PubMed—indexed for MEDLINE].

11. A. T. Kamilova, N. N. Akhmedov, D. B. Pulatova, B.
    A. Nurmatov.
    [Intestinal microbiocenosis in children with intestinal
    enzymopathy] Zh Mikrobiol Epidemiol Immunobiol.
    3 (May–Jun 2001):97–9. Russian. PMID: 11550576
    [PubMed—indexed for MEDLINE].

12. J. Kocian.
[Lactobacilli in the treatment of dyspepsia due
to dysmicrobia of various causes] Vnitr Lek.
40(2) (Feb 1994):79–83. Czech. PMID: 8140765
[PubMed—indexed for MEDLINE].

13. M. J. Hopkins, R. Sharp, G. T. Macfarlane.
Age and disease related changes in intestinal
bacterial populations assessed by cell culture, 16S
rRNA abundance, and community cellular fatty acid
profiles. Gut. 48(2) (Feb 2001):198–205. PMID:
11156640 [PubMed—indexed for MEDLINE].

14. P. Sirakov, I. Dimov.
[Bacterial intestinal microflora of patients with a
constipation syndrome] Vutr Boles. 20(4)(1981):
24–28. Bulgarian. PMID: 7303637 [PubMed—
indexed for MEDLINE].

15. G. Zoppi, M. Cinquetti, A. Luciano, A. Benini, A.
Muner, E. Bertazzoni Minelli.
The intestinal ecosystem in chronic functional
constipation. Acta Paediatr. 87(8)(Aug 1998):
836–841. PMID: 9736230 [PubMed—indexed
for MEDLINE].

16. J. N. Kenyon.
Food sensitivity, a search for underlying causes.
Case study of 12 patients. Acupunct Electrother
Res. 11(1)(1986):1–13. PMID: 2872775 [PubMed—
indexed for MEDLINE].

17. M. Knoke, H. Bernhardt.
Clinical significance of changes of flora in the
upper digestive tract. Infection. 17(4)(Jul-Aug
1989):255–258. PMID: 2767770 [PubMed—indexed
for MEDLINE].

18. P. R. Cordts, M. V. Kaminski, S. Raju, M. R. Clark,
K. M. Woo.
Could gut-liver function derangements cause
chronic venous insufficiency? Vasc Surg. (Mar-
Apr 2001): 107–114. PMID: 11668378 [PubMed—
indexed for MEDLINE].

19. P. M. Kidd.
Attention deficit/hyperactivity disorder (ADHD) in
children: rationale for its integrative management.
Altern Med Rev. 5(5) (Oct 2000):402–28.
Review. PMID: 11056411 [PubMed—indexed
for MEDLINE].

20. Archives of Family Medicine, 52(6):593-6 1996 Nov-Dec

21. European Journal of Clinical Nutrition, 52(6):436-40 1998 June

22. British Medical Journal January 27, 2001;322:210-212.

23. American Journal of Clinical Nutrition 2003; 77:600-604.

24. A. Hirazumi & E. Furusawa, National Library of Medicine website: Phytother Res, 13(5)(Aug 1999): 380–387; www.ncbi.nlm.nih.gov, cited 13 May 2002.

25. Ann NY Academy of Science, 2001 Dec: 952: 161–168 National Library of Medicine website: www.ncbi.nlm.nih.gov; Cancer preventive effect of *Morinda citrifolia* by M. Y. Wang, C. Su; cited 13 May 2002.

26. T. Hiramatsu; M. Imoto; et al; Noni Research; Anti-Cancer Activity; Cancer Letters 73, 161–166(1993); website: www.incc.org; cited 13 May 2002.

27. C. Younos; A. Rolland; et al; Noni Research; Anti-Cancer Activity; Planta Medica , Oct; 56, 430–

434(1990): website: www.ncbi.nlm.nih.gov; cited
13 May 2002.

28. S. Banerjee; A.D. Johnson; et al; Noni Research;
American Journal of Chinese Medicine,
2006;34(3):503-509 website: www.ncbi.nlmlnih.
gov: cited 17 July 2006.

29. S.W. Kim; B.K. Jeong; et al; Noni Research; Journal
of Medicinal Food. 2005 Winter;8(4):552-5 website:
www.ncbi.nlm.nih.gov: cited 17 July 2006.

30. C.J. Jensen; J. Westendor; et al; Noni Juice Protects
the Liver; European Journal of Gastroenterology
& Hepatology. Volume 18(5) May 2006:575-577
website: www.eurojgh.com: cited 17 July 2006.

31. Neil Solomon, M.D., Ph.D., *The Noni Phenomenon*,
Direct Source Publishing, 1999, pp. 48 & 51.

32. Ralph M. Heinicke, Ph.D., *The Xeronine System*,
Direct Source Publishing, 2001; pp. 19–64.

33. National Library of Medicine Website: www.ncbi.nlm.
nih.gov; Phytother Res; A. Hirazumi & E. Furusawa,
13(5)(Aug 1999): 380–387; cited 13 May 2002.

INDEX

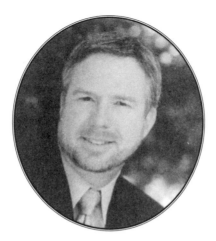

ABOUT THE AUTHOR

Richard L. Becker, D.O. is the co-host of the national television health talk show, *Your Health with Dr. Richard and Cindy Becker*. He is widely recognized as an expert on health supplements and holistic healing methods. He is board certified in Family Practice and Osteopathic Manipulative Therapy. He is a graduate of the University of Health Sciences, College of Osteopathic Medicine, Kansas City, Missouri, and of the Loma Linda University, Riverside, California, where he received his Bachelor of Arts degree in biochemistry. His twenty-two years of experience in medicine, treating the whole body, brings a unique brand of practicality and insight to family practice. Dr. Becker currently resides in North Central Texas with his wife, Cindy, and their two adult daughters.

CONTACT INFORMATION

BIO INNOVATIONS
PO Box 2485
Rockwall, Texas 75087

888.442.6161
www.bioinnovations.net
www.alohanoni.com